EAT CHO
DRINK ALCOHOL
AND BE LEAN AND
HEALTHY

Andrew Jobling

HINKLER
BOOKS

How to Have Balance, Enjoy Your Life and Achieve Great Things

- Learn how to create long-term change while still enjoying your indulgences.
- Understand the powerful effect of food on your body and mind.
- Learn how to control blood sugar levels and live a longer, leaner, more energised life.
- Learn simple strategies to help you to achieve what you have previously thought unattainable.

Cover Design: Sam Grimmer

Eat Chocolate, Drink Alcohol and be Lean and Healthy
Published in 2004 by Hinkler Books Pty Ltd
17–23 Redwood Drive
Dingley VIC 3172 Australia
www.hinklerbooks.com

Text: © Andrew Jobling 2004
Design: © Hinkler Books Pty Ltd 2004

Reprinted 2004, 2005

ISBN 1 7412 1512 9
Printed and bound in China

Acknowledgments

I would like to thank the following people:

Sally Jobling – for her contribution to the recipes and ongoing love, support and great dinners.

Sue Jobling – for the inspiration to keep going when things got tough.

Bill Jobling – for never letting anything get under the radar.

Craig Harper – for always being a great lead.

Kumara Lord – for her influence on my beliefs and understanding.

Terry Martinez – for helping to formulate my beliefs and understanding of nutrition.

Gemma Horsfield – for her indepth knowledge of chocolate.

Jo Fleischer – for helping under difficult circumstances.

Hinkler Books and Steve Ungar – for having enough faith in me to publish this book.

All of my clients – for helping me to learn.

All of my work colleagues and business associates – for being great to work with and learn from, and for being a positive influence.

CONTENTS

Introduction

Life is precious, so why do we treat ourselves as if we are replaceable? Stop and think for a moment how precious your life really is. Think about how easily it could be taken from you and think about how much you take for granted.

Consider your life at this moment. Are you busy? Do you skip meals? Do you eat food for convenience or for health? Do you smoke? Do you drink too much alcohol, caffeine or soft drinks? Have you dieted? How many times? Do you feel stressed at times? Do you eat a balanced variety of foods? Do you enjoy eating or does it create extra stress? Do you understand the effect of all these things on your health, wellbeing and longevity?

Did you know that about 80 percent of health problems such as being overweight or obese, diabetes, heart disease and cancer could be avoided by the lifestyle choices we make and the way we choose to live?[1]

Would you like to be able to enjoy chocolate, alcohol and other indulgences and still be leaner, more energised, less stressed, happier and live longer? Do you think it is possible? I am here to tell you that it is. So who am I?

I am a qualified personal trainer and co-director at Harper's Personal Training Pty Ltd, Melbourne, Australia. I am a founding director of Twist Pty Ltd, Melbourne, Australia, a company dedicated to educating people about the amazing positive effect of eating the right type of food at

[1] *The Daily Telegraph* (3/7/00), p85 'Survival Instincts'

the right time of day, and I am currently working as an educator, motivator and life changer.

Since the 1980s I have been a teacher of physical education, a gym instructor, a personal trainer and a public speaker. In that time I have worked with and spoken to thousands of people with the aim of helping them to improve their looks, health and the quality of every aspect of their lives.

I am passionate about helping others achieve their potential. I believe in the awesome power of food. I have experienced and seen the positive effects good eating can have on health, energy, body (size, shape and image), performance and self-confidence. I love helping others create balance and long-term change.

My knowledge and passion about food and its effects has not come from years of study. It has come from years of experience, trial and error, reading, listening and talking to people with knowledge I didn't then have. It came from refining ideas, concepts and theories that were continually changing and will continue to do so. Most of all it came from practice and the understanding that everyone is different and that for every single person the plan for success will vary.

As a footballer for the St Kilda Football Club in the Australian Football League in my teens and early 20s, I wondered why I never really achieved what I'd hoped for. I spent seven years at St Kilda and only played 24 senior games until my career was terminated by the club when I was age 23. I chose to play amateur football for the remainder of my career and as I learned more and gained some wisdom about food and training I achieved more than I thought possible.

As an inexperienced gym instructor and personal trainer I often wondered why my clients never really got the results they were after, considering the amount of training they were doing. The old cliché really rings true: 'If only I knew then what I know now!'

The incredibly positive long-term effects that I've had on the lives of the countless people I've worked with is testament to the value of my accumulated knowledge. However, I still get frustrated because I can't reach as many people as I would like – there are only so many hours in the day. That is where this book comes in.

Eat Chocolate, Drink Alcohol and be Lean and Healthy reflects a way of life and the importance of balance in all areas of life. I hope to help you understand that getting in shape doesn't mean giving up all the foods that you enjoy. By following a realistic, consistent and enjoyable plan there is room for indulgence while you keep improving your health, body shape and quality of life.

I hope you enjoy reading about my passion. It may even change your life, as it did mine.

Part 1

The Objectives

1
Slow Down

Why is everyone in such a hurry to lose weight, get fit and look and feel fantastic? Well, I guess the answer to this question is pretty obvious. Probably the more relevant question is how many people do you know who have made long-term life changes in less than eight weeks and maintained those changes?

Before you decide to try and change something about yourself in eight weeks, stop and think about how long it took to get to the point where you decided it was time to take action to change. I am guessing it would be more than eight weeks!

If you were to add up all the short-term life changing attempts you have made, what would be the total time you have devoted to this pursuit? Are you in any better shape now than you were when you began the first attempt? If you are, then maybe you don't need to read any further. If you are no better off, or even worse, then this chapter is vital for you to digest (pardon the pun).

The bottom line is that it is not possible to make huge life changes in a short time and expect to maintain them. Anyone who tries is setting themselves up for failure, yet many people will do it time and time again. A diet here, a cream there, a piece of fitness equipment that is more useful as a clothes horse, a fitness regime that lasts two weeks, a pill that promises to reduce cellulite but just reduces your bank balance and many more wonderful ideas and scams that promise everything and deliver only heartache and another failed attempt.

It is time that we stopped looking for an easy, quick way to get into shape and understood that long-term results require time, effort and consistency. But even more important than getting the results you desire, is that you enjoy the journey.

Ask yourself this question the next time you attempt to lose fat or get in shape: **'Do I enjoy and can I maintain this process long term (i.e. forever)?'** If the answer is yes then you are on the right track. If the answer is no, then don't even try it, because chances are it won't last and eventually you will be back or behind where you are now.

The secret is to slow down. Don't try to change everything in one week. If it takes you 12 months to slowly redevelop your behaviours and habits and you then maintain them for the rest of your life then it has been one year well spent. One year out of your whole life is a pretty small sacrifice, especially if it changes it for the better forever. I am assuming that, like me, you want to live to at least 120!

On the other hand if you lose 10kg (22lb) in six weeks, but then put 12kg (26lb) back on in the next 10 weeks not only have you wasted 16 weeks of your life (in terms of your body) and have an extra 2kg (4lb) to lose, but the psychological scarring that occurs through your perceived lack of discipline will have far-reaching effects on your self esteem.

A very important point needs to be made here: **when you can't maintain a diet, it is the diet that has failed, NOT you.**

Don't try to give up all the food you like because you think it is bad for you. You should be able to enjoy chocolate, alcohol, pizza or whatever your favourite indulgence is, in moderation.

Pick one or two aspects of your life that need to change, then take the time to change and re-establish habits. For example if you don't eat breakfast and the only change you make is to eat something as soon as you get up you will notice positive results almost immediately. Once that has been successful choose another one or two areas and do the same. It would be wise to employ the help of a professional, personal trainer, mentor or someone you trust to assist you through this vital process.

Case Study: Gloria and Roberta

The following is a true story. Names have been changed to protect the privacy of the individuals.

Two potential clients, Gloria and Roberta, came to me at about the same time. They came independently of each other and had the same goal: to lose weight to fit into dresses for the Spring Horse Racing Carnival. They both wanted to lose 8–10kg (18–22lb) in five weeks.

I gave them the same advice. Forget about trying to lose all that weight quickly for this carnival; instead, spend the next 12 months getting ready for the next spring carnival and every spring carnival after that.

Gloria wasn't happy with that plan and so we parted ways. I referred her to a trainer who could help with her goal. Roberta, on the other hand, was sick of yoyo dieting and wanted to make some long-term changes. We got started on changing her life forever.

From all reports Gloria looked great at the premier race meeting that year, having lost 8kg to fit into her size eight outfit.

Roberta was looking good, not exactly how she would have liked, but she had the bigger picture in mind. By the spring carnival one year later she looked stunning and felt fantastic. She had made some significant changes to her thinking and behaviours over the 12-month period and was now reaping the rewards. She had lost significant fat and was still losing it, she had great energy and had never felt or looked better. Now, she will never go back to the way she was.

To my knowledge, Gloria was back with the same personal trainer exactly 12 months after I had first met her with the same desperate goal, except this year she had more weight to lose. She was and is riding the body weight rollercoaster and will continue to do so until she decides to change her thinking.

The fantastic long-term process that Roberta undertook relied on the following:

- You need to eat regularly to have more energy, lose fat and perform better. This may be significantly more food than you are used to.

- Training more won't necessarily lead to quicker results.

- Your weight is not an indicator of fat loss.

- Alcohol, chocolate and take-away food in moderation will not negatively affect your progress. In fact, if you know you can have indulgences, the process will be more enjoyable.

- Consistency is the key.

- The first thing you will notice is an increase in energy levels.

- Have faith in yourself. You can achieve anything you want – just give yourself a chance.

What is more important to you?

1 Getting results quickly and sacrificing the way you feel, the food you enjoy and doing the things you love for a look that you can't maintain. Or . . .

2 Taking the time to re-establish routines, habits and behaviours, feeling fantastic, enjoying eating, performing better in all aspects, achieving the look you want and increasing the quality of your life forever.

If the first option is your preference then read no further. This book is not for you. If number 2 sounds good then read on.

A Brief History

Since the 1970s there have been enormous changes in our attitudes to food, health, nutrition and wellbeing. Two of the most significant events that stand out in my mind in terms of their catalytic effect on our general health and wellbeing today are:

1 The gym and weight loss revolution.

2 The explosion of the career obsessive, 'I need it done yesterday', no-time, high-stress generation.

In terms of the first factor, I have one question to ask. If over the last 25–30 years we have been more conscious of exercise and healthy eating, why are we more overweight than we have ever been? Furthermore, why is the incidence of heart disease, diabetes, stroke and cancer at its highest?

One of the most obvious contributors is lifestyle. As a nation we started to work longer hours than ever. The introduction of mobile phones, faxes, emails and the internet changed expectations about how quickly we could complete tasks. As demands from employers increased we devoted less time to exercise, appropriate eating, leisure activities and laughter.

Food convenience became a priority and consequently myriad products and services were born. Think about all the fast food outlets and convenience products that have sprung up like mushrooms all over the country. Let's be honest: how easy is it to drive through and get a burger and fries or reach into your bag for a muesli bar or packet of chips when you are rushed?

During this period, while the technology of food supply and convenience products was advancing, our basic knowledge of nutrition was only just evolving. The main aim of food companies was to make products that tasted better, looked better and lasted longer than their competition and that were safe from contamination. Unfortunately they did not foresee the dire health effects that this processing could potentially create.

To make products taste better, fat was added (a potentially dangerous synthetic fat, which I will expand on in Chapter 5).

To make products safe from contamination they were pasteurised and/or heated, destroying many of the valuable nutrients.

Increasing the shelf life and look of products required preservatives and other additives. In small amounts these may not be harmful, but in large amounts and over extended periods the possible effects include increased risk of heart disease, diabetes, stroke, cancer, kidney failure and other common health disorders.

Many food products were also treated with artificial flavourings and sugars, which in large amounts and over extended periods may also be detrimental to health.

Losing fat was becoming an even greater priority for people. Many gyms came in and went out of business. Why? Because it didn't happen quickly enough – people weren't prepared to spend the time or the effort to do what it took for long-term results.

Many people didn't and maybe still don't understand the difference between fat loss and weight loss. They placed far too much attention and effort on losing weight and what the scales told them without realising that it is fat loss which is the key. **Fat loss may not be associated with significant weight loss and just because weight is not decreasing does not mean that fat isn't.** This is an area that I will cover in more detail as we proceed.

Then came the array of weight loss organisations and the promise of quick weight loss – but would it last? And who could forget liposuction, fat loss tablets, body wrapping, diet after diet, and myriad equipment for fast, effortless weight loss? We kept trying and trying, but continually and painfully found ourselves back at square one!

In the supermarket we were overjoyed to see a number of low-fat or fat-free products appear on the shelves. It seemed too good to be true – low fat chips, fat free salad dressings, 98 percent fat free rice crackers, 100 percent fat free jelly-beans, low-fat ice cream etc. They were low fat **and** tasted good – something had to be wrong.

Something **was** wrong. We were still getting fatter, more stressed and experiencing more disease and other ailments than ever.

What we didn't and are still struggling to realise is that although a product may be low in fat, if it is high in sugar and other highly refined and artificial ingredients, the effect is just as damaging to the body. Look at the ingredients of a popular low-fat breakfast bar and see if you can count how many forms of sugar and refined and artificial ingredients are present. What is the number one ingredient in fat-free salad dressing? Sugar. What is the number one ingredient of low-fat ice cream? Sugar.

Why do we keep going back for all these products? Because they are marketed very cleverly, we think they are good for us and we are addicted to the sugar and refined carbohydrates they contain.

Why do we keep going back to diets, fat loss organisations, and quick weight loss schemes? I believe that it's because we are too busy and don't have the time to find out and do what is required. We are continually searching for and hoping for one of these products to live up to their promises and actually provide us with the long-term results we have been striving, hoping and grasping for.

It's now time to get off the rollercoaster. Stop, learn and apply sensible long-term strategies to achieve everything you desire. Not just for tomorrow, not for next week, not even next month, but for next year and every year for the rest of your life.

Supporting Reference

Pilzer, P., *The Wellness Revolution* (2002), John Wiley and Sons, USA.

2
The Carbohydrate Phenomenon

The crucial questions I hear every day of my working life include:

How do I lose weight? How do I feel better? How do I get more energy? How do I prevent disease? How do I live longer?

Every person you speak to will give you their theory on eating:

'Eat no carbohydrates after 2pm.'

'Eat only fruit until lunchtime.'

'Don't eat grapes, they are full of sugar.'

'Carbohydrates make you fat.'

'Protein makes you fat.'

'Cut all fat out of your diet.'

'It's okay to drink vodka because it has no calories.'

. . . and a million other statements.

The big question is: who do you believe? I can't tell you who to believe. All I will say is make sure that whoever you decide to listen to makes sense and that you are comfortable with the lifestyle they suggest. In this book, I will present you with another theory, one which I hope does make sense and which you feel you can embrace. Let's talk some details.

All food is made up of one or more of six nutrients:

1 Carbohydrates

2 Proteins

3 Fats (or lipids)

4 Vitamins

5 Minerals

6 Water.

Each of these nutrients plays different and vital roles in the efficient functioning of the body and prevention of disease. I will talk more about all the nutrients as we progress, but I want to devote this chapter to helping you develop a sound awareness of carbohydrates.

Carbohydrates

We have turned 360 degrees in our thinking about carbohydrates. There was a time when carbohydrates were the 'be
all and end all', and vital for health and losing fat. More
recently they have been labelled as the reason why we are
getting fatter and less healthy. The famous 'carbohydrate-free
diet' is commonplace. In two years there will be another fad.
We will discuss diets and fads in Chapter 12.

Carbohydrates are an essential part of a long-term, life-
changing eating plan. However, because carbohydrates are
misunderstood, they receive bad press. Here's where people
go wrong:

1 They are eating the wrong types of carbohydrates. That is,
   carbohydrates that are highly processed, nutrient deficient and high in sugar and other artificial ingredients.

2 They are not eating carbohydrates when they need them,
   and are eating far too many when they don't.

**The secret is to eat the right carbohydrates at the right
time of day.** Before we get too far into this extremely important area, we need to learn more about the varying effects of
different carbohydrates.

Carbohydrates and Blood Sugar Levels

Each nutrient contained in food is vital to our long-term health and enjoyment. But when it comes to energy, carbohydrate is our body's preferred source.

Carbohydrates are found in a wide range of foods from bread, rice, pasta, potatoes, cereals, and fruits and vegetables to lollies, desserts and many soft and sweet drinks. Some carbohydrates are highly processed and refined, others are more natural, wholegrain and complex. Different carbohydrates have varying effects on the body.

You may have heard or will hear a blanket statement about carbohydrates, such as: 'Carbohydrates make you fat'. This is a simplified and misleading comment. It would only be true where the wrong type of carbohydrates were consumed at the least appropriate time of the day on an ongoing basis.

When you eat a food that contains carbohydrate, your body breaks the carbohydrate component down to its most basic form. That is glucose or sugar. It may be hard to believe, but when you are holding a potato or loaf of bread you are basically holding sugar!

This sugar enters the bloodstream and consequently the body's blood sugar levels begin to rise. Every carbohydrate is different and will be broken down to sugar at a different rate. The rate at which a carbohydrate is broken down to sugar determines the amount of sugar released into the blood and hence the rate at which the blood sugar levels rise.

For example, let's take two pieces of bread: a slice of white and a slice of 100 percent rye. The white bread, being made of highly refined white flour, will break down and be converted to sugar rapidly. The rye bread made from more complex rye flour will take a considerably longer time to break down to sugar (see graph 1).

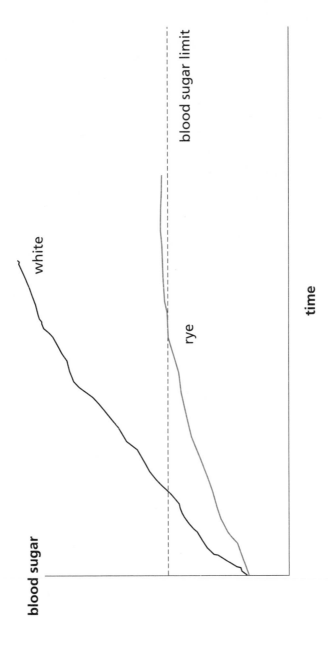

Graph 1 Sugar release into the blood for white and rye bread

Too Much Blood Sugar

Regardless of the type of carbohydrate eaten, immediately after sugar enters the bloodstream the pancreas releases a small amount of the hormone insulin. Insulin's job is to regulate blood sugar levels and make sure they don't go too high. If, however, in the case of the white bread where blood sugar levels rise rapidly, beyond the blood's sugar limit, the body's response is much more dramatic.

The pancreas responds by releasing large amounts of insulin to cope with the blood sugar excess. The insulin attaches itself to sugar molecules and transports them to be stored outside the blood. The muscles and liver cells receive the first storage of sugar, which will be converted to energy and used when needed.

The storage capacity of the muscle cells and liver cells is limited and may also be inhibited by damaged cell membranes resulting from a diet high in processed foods and synthetic fats (refer to Chapter 5). This means there will be an excess of sugar in the blood. This excess will be stored as fat, and will continue to do so as there is no limit as to how much your fat cells can store.

It is interesting to note at this point that food need contain no fat to create the situation described above. We are regularly tricked by clever marketing into buying products that contain little or no fat. The supermarket shelves are full of these products that the consumer buys and eats with delight in the knowledge that if it's low in fat it has got to be good. Not so.

What we are not told is that the majority of these products contain many highly refined sugars, carbohydrates and fats in addition to artificial additives used to replace the taste lost when the major fat source is removed. The effect of these ingredients creates the situation we are specifically trying to avoid by eating them.

In addition to fat storage, excess insulin negatively affects health in other ways. An excess of insulin causes an increase in the production of bad (LDL) cholesterol (see Chapter 5), an increase in blood pressure and a dramatic drop in blood sugar levels. This drop causes fatigue and many other symptoms and side effects, creating a greater likelihood of the same type of food being eaten again to rapidly raise blood sugar levels once more. This is a time when you may experience a craving for chocolate or other food (see graph 2).

It would be fair to say that your blood sugar level reflects your energy level. When your blood sugar levels are high, energy levels are good. When low, feelings of lethargy and irritability are prevalent.

As a result of this rapid blood sugar level drop you may experience any or all of the following:

• Fatigue and lethargy

• Moodiness and irritability

• A reduced ability to concentrate

• A strong urge or craving for sweet food

• A lack of ability to make the wisest food choice (due to point 4) and the risk of eating for the sake of eating.

In this state of low blood sugar a common response is to eat carbohydrates that will rapidly replace the energy lacking.

How many times have you felt any of the above symptoms and eaten lollies, soft drink or other food in order to give you that quick blood sugar hit? It certainly works! Blood sugar will rise quickly – until the insulin kicks in again and sends it plummeting. This may occur continuously each day.

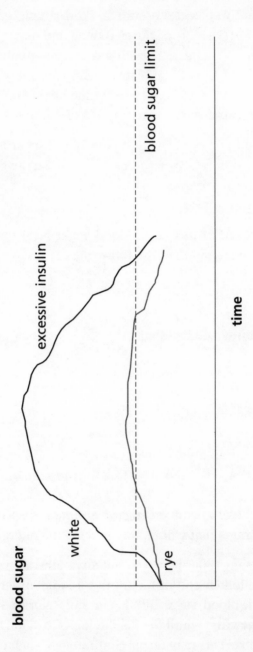

Graph 2 Overall effect on blood sugar of white and rye bread

This is a trap that many people get themselves into on a daily basis, one that they feel unable to escape from. Their food intake is controlled by the blood sugar rollercoaster, and consequently so is every aspect of their life (see graph 3).

This continual feeling of being out of control has many long-term, negative psychological, physical and emotional effects that will be discussed as we progress.

In addition to the continual daily highs and lows of energy, mood and performance the long-term effects of continual spikes and falls of blood sugar are significant. There is strong evidence to confirm that these eating habits, over a period of time, contribute to negative health conditions such as; obesity, heart disease and type II diabetes, just to name a few.

Low Blood Sugar Levels

The blood sugar rollercoaster is reasonably common for many people.

Are you a person who is always rushed, skips breakfast, misses morning snacks and drinks a lot of coffee? Do you work long hours (at home or work)? Do you exercise or attempt to exercise regularly? Do you eat only two to three times a day? Do you feel lethargic most of the time? Do you crave sugar, chocolate or other foods in the afternoon and evening?

If you answer yes to the majority of these questions, then you are in good company and your blood sugar levels quite possibly resemble graph 4.

I would estimate that 90 percent of the people I speak to have low blood sugar levels on a continual basis. These people include:

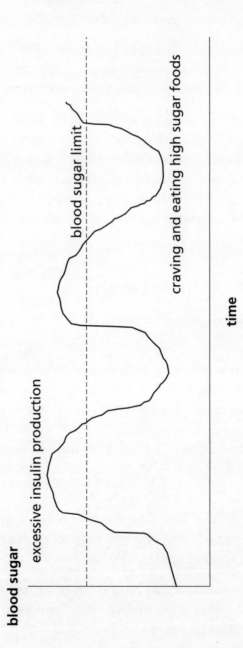

Graph 3 The blood sugar rollercoaster

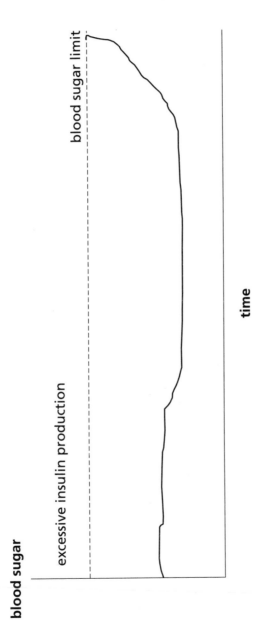

Graph 4 Low blood sugar levels

- Busy career people

- Busy family minded people

- People on calorie- or carbohydrate-restricted diets

- People scared that eating too much will make them fat

- People who don't fully understand the enormous benefits of eating regularly

- People who have undesirable eating patterns and habits.

Here are the many negative effects of low blood sugar, especially when low blood sugar is experienced over extended periods:

- Lethargy

- Reduced ability to concentrate

- Reduced motivation and ability to exercise

- Moodiness and irritability

- Uncontrollable emotions

- Regular cravings

- Poor eating choices

- Guilt associated with the response to these cravings

- Tendency to binge and the possibility of eating disorders

- Emotional decisions as opposed to logical ones

- Lower quality relationships

- Reduced ability to deal with stresses.

These are some symptoms that you may notice every day if your blood sugars are too low. But what about the less obvious, yet highly significant effects that you may not be aware of. Think about the reason why we eat. The most basic, essential reason for eating is to give us energy. What is our body supposed to do for energy if we are not supplying it with enough for our daily requirements?

The common theory is that by reducing calories and/or carbohydrates from your plan you will force your body to activate fat stores as an alternative energy source.

Unfortunately this theory has some flaws. It is true that your body will use some fat as an alternative energy supply. However, your body is only willing to give up so much fat when it reaches a state of 'famine' (or extended calorie restriction). Sooner or later, your body will hang on to your fat stores for long-term survival.

This leaves us with the same problem: if there is not enough energy coming in, and your body is hanging on to fat, then where do we get the energy to get through the day? Your body is very smart and will do what it has to do to keep you alive and it doesn't care how you look or feel. It will now begin to break down lean muscle and covert it to usable energy. For people dieting and trying to lose weight this would seem like a good thing, because the scales will be going the right way.

What they are failing to realise is that this weight they are losing is largely muscle and water, NOT fat. Every gram of carbohydrate contains 3 grams of water, so you can imagine how much weight will disappear quickly when carbohydrates are reduced or eliminated from our eating plan.

The consequence of losing muscle is a reduction in metabolism (the rate at which your body functions, including fat burning). The long-term effect of a slow metabolism is a reduced ability to burn fat and therefore a much greater chance of storing significantly more fat than before, if and when calorie intake returns to a sustainable level.

Other long-term effects of extended calorie/carbohydrate restriction include:

- Affected brain function

- Possible brain damage

- Possibility of liver damage and disease

- Decreased contraction of the heart.

Well, I've convinced myself! The final critical effect of this type of under-eating during the day is the insatiable appetite it causes in the afternoon and evening.

Is dinner your largest meal of the day? Do you eat more from 4 to 9pm (five hours) than you do from 7am to 4pm (nine hours)? During which of these periods are you more active (either physically or mentally)?

Consider these questions, and then think about what your body would do with pre-dinner nibbles, a large bowl of pasta, dessert and a post-dinner snack.

What do you do after dinner? If you are like 90 percent of the population and myself you sit on the couch, watch TV or read and then go to bed. What do you think your body does with all that food you have just eaten? After a lengthy and energy-consuming digestion, which will most likely affect your night's sleep, the majority of the food will most likely be stored as fat.

Okay, so we know that blood sugar levels that are too high or too low have major implications for our health

What is the solution? The solution lies in the ability to control our blood sugar levels. The blood sugar objective is looked at in detail in the next chapter.

3
The Blood Sugar Objective

The ability to control our blood sugar levels is vital. If we can elevate them to an optimal level and then maintain them there for the day, on a consistent basis, we go a long way to achieving long-term success.

If we can achieve the scenario represented by graph 5 then anything is possible.

- We will have optimal energy (all day)

- We will concentrate better and consequently be more productive

- We will be more motivated to exercise

- We will exercise more effectively (eg, run faster, lift heavier, go for longer)

- We will have more consistent moods

- We will crave less (craving is largely a symptom of low blood sugar)

- We will make sensible eating choices

- We will not overeat in the evening

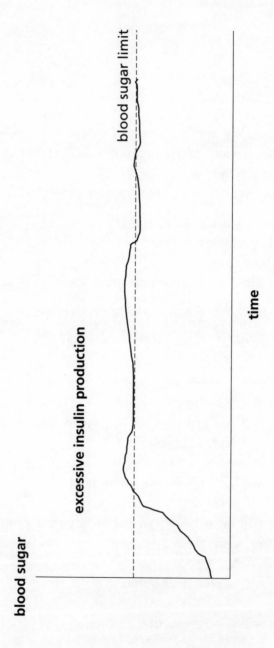

Graph 5 Optimal level of blood sugar in the body, through the day

- We will enjoy our indulgences in moderation without negative physical or emotional effects

- We will get leaner, fitter and stronger

- We will be healthier

- We will have better relationships with the important people in our lives

- We will achieve greater things in all areas

- We will live a longer, more fulfilling, more balanced and enjoyable life.

Sounds pretty good, doesn't it? Believe me it is possible and all it requires is some understanding, some organisation, consistency and a true belief in yourself.

I will provide you with the understanding and some strategies; the rest is up to you. I urge you to make the effort as the rewards are incredible.

Glycemic Index

Okay, so we know the aim is to raise blood sugar levels to the blood sugar limit and then keep them around there for the day. How do we do this and how do we know where this level is?

Let me answer the latter question first. The broken line on the graph (page 41) represents the optimal level of sugar in the blood above which an excess of insulin will be produced, and below which a lack of energy will result. It is different for everyone. A good indication that we have reached this level is when we notice a more consistent energy level, an even temperament and an absence of cravings – and this may take some trial and error.

Okay, so how do we get our blood sugars up, and how do we maintain them? The first step is to have an understanding of Glycemic Index.

Have you heard of the Glycemic Index? If not, it doesn't matter because you are about to learn all about it. From now on I will refer to it as GI. As I mentioned in Chapter 2, every time you eat a food that contains carbohydrates your body will break it down to sugar or glucose. The rate at which this happens and the amount of glucose released into the bloodstream depends on the type and amount of food.

The old way of thinking about this involved the terms 'complex' and 'simple' carbohydrates. Complex carbohydrates were considered to break down to glucose over time and provide a slow release of sugar into the bloodstream. They include foods such as pasta, potatoes, rice, pumpkin, bread, cereals. Simple carbohydrates were considered to be all those that break down quickly and release sugar rapidly into the bloodstream causing a quick energy rush, such as lollies, soft drinks, chocolate. Then the GI came along to really throw this understanding into chaos.

Each carbohydrate-containing food was laboratory tested and its effect on blood sugar measured. Pure glucose was thought to have the greatest effect on blood sugar and was set at a value of 100 (its Glycemic Index). Every other food was then measured against glucose and a relative GI calculated. The results surprised a lot of people.

What follows is a very basic Glycemic Index (a more detailed one appears in the Appendix):

FOOD	GLYCEMIC INDEX
Beer (maltose)	105
Glucose	100
Parsnip	97
Rice pasta	92
Rice cakes/crackers	87
Rice	85 (av)
Potatoes	80 (av)
Lollies (average)	80
Cornflakes	80
Pumpkin	75
White/wholemeal bread	70 (av)
Table sugar	60
Basmati rice	57
Doongara rice	56
Natural muesli	55 (av)
Long grain rice	50
100% rye bread	50
Sweet potato	50
Plain chocolate	45
Oats	42
Low fat yoghurt	30
Fructose	23
Soy and linseed bread	36
Green vegetables	15 or less
Fresh meat, chicken, fish and egg	negligible
Fats and oils	negligible

In practical terms, what do these numbers mean?

Foods with a high GI (above 65) will be converted to glucose rapidly, causing a large amount of sugar to enter the bloodstream. Consequently, it is likely that blood sugar levels will rise rapidly resulting in a substantial insulin response. The results of which have been discussed in Chapter 2.

Foods with a moderate GI (50–65) cause a more gradual release of glucose into the bloodstream. This causes blood sugar levels to rise more gradually and last longer.

Foods with a low GI (less than 50) will maintain blood sugar levels as they are. As the GI gets even lower, the effect on blood sugar levels decreases due to low carbohydrate content and a slow rate of sugar release into the blood. Refer to graph 6 (next page).

Generally speaking we should eat low to moderate GI foods to maintain a stable level of blood sugar. There are, however, times when a high GI food is the best option. This will be discussed in detail in later chapters.

It is interesting to note that some of the high GI foods are ones we have considered to be complex carbohydrates. For example: rice, potatoes, white and brown bread, pumpkin.

Who would have thought that a potato would have a more dramatic effect on blood sugar than jellybeans? Certainly not I! Who would have thought that beer could send your blood sugars through the roof! Many a tear has been shed over this realisation!

The GI values raise many questions, such as:

1 Why is the GI of long grain rice so much lower than other rice varieties?

2 Why is sweet potato lower than potato and pumpkin?

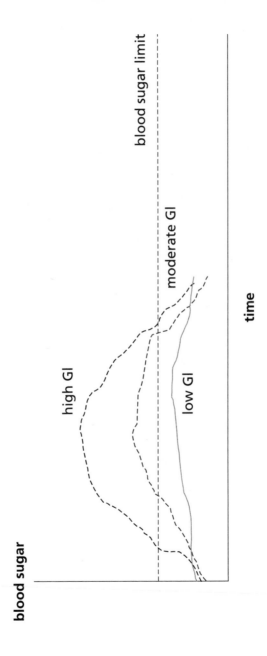

Graph 6 The effect of GI levels on blood sugar

3 How can chocolate have such a low GI?

4 What's the story with parsnip?

5 How can beer be higher than glucose?

6 Why are meat and fats so low?

I'm sure that you have many more questions, which hopefully will be answered as we progress. First, I will explain the above queries:

1 The GI value refers to how quickly a food is converted to glucose. This in turn is related to the food's chemical make-up. All carbohydrates are compounds of carbon, hydrogen and oxygen bonded together. Each carbohydrate compound is different in terms of the strength and complexity of the bond. Long grain rice has a much more complex bond of carbon, hydrogen and oxygen and therefore it takes longer to break down.

2 Sweet potato has a lower GI for the same reason.

3 While chocolate has a high sugar content, it is also made up of a significant percentage of fat. Fat being a low GI substance (as I will discuss later) will reduce or negate the effect of the high GI ingredients. This may seem to be good news for a lot of people, but don't get too excited!

4 The good news about parsnip is that most people don't like it anyway so its GI is irrelevant! I apologise to those people who are parsnip fans. As you read further you will get some ideas about how to still enjoy your parsnip without your blood sugar levels rocketing through the roof.

5   Beer is made primarily from a carbohydrate, or sugar, called maltose. Remember the test substance was glucose and all other carbohydrates were measured against it. When beer/malt was tested, its effect on blood sugar levels was found to be greater than glucose.

6   Protein foods are very low or negligible when it comes to GI. When you think about this, it makes sense – how many carbohydrates are in a chicken breast fillet? None, so why would it have a GI when this is a measure of carbohydrate absorption? Fats and oils have a low GI for the same reason. Including proteins and good fats with your meals is a great way to reduce overall GI of the meal, not to mention the other benefits of foods containing these components.

Some of the above questions raise even further issues. It is not often that we would eat a single food by itself. I mean how many people eat a slice of white bread and nothing else? And not many people would sit down on the couch and settle into a good movie with a baked parsnip to munch on!

The fact that we often combine single foods and ingredients to come up with our meals is a good thing, in terms of GI. Some food combinations, however, may have a detrimental effect on digestion, but we will discuss this at a later stage.

In terms of GI, when we combine different foods the overall GI of the meal is, very simply put, an average of the individual ingredients. It is not quite this simple, but I hope you get the idea.

Let's say for example you want to make yourself a sandwich, but you only have white bread. We know that white bread has a high GI of 70, is highly processed and probably not the very best choice. It is possible to eat and enjoy this white bread on occasions and ensure that this sandwich is low GI at the same time. It's all to do with what you put in the sandwich. If you spread some avocado on the bread (avocado being higher in fat will have a low GI), add some low GI salad such as lettuce, cucumber, tomato, and some lean chicken you will significantly reduce the overall GI of the sandwich.

By making sure that you always include some protein, healthy fats and other natural, low GI ingredients with each meal you will ensure that its GI is one that will help control blood sugars and sustain energy.

At this point I must caution against an excitable frenzy towards high fat foods (particularly synthetic and saturated fat) just because they have a low GI. Excess dietary fat will be stored as fat by the body far more readily than excess blood sugar, even though it has a low GI. I will talk about fats in more detail in Chapter 5.

Dietary Fibre

With controlling blood sugar in mind, the best types of carbohydrates are those in their natural state. These are carbohydrates high in dietary fibre. Dietary fibre is the part of the plant that cannot be digested when eaten. Insufficient dietary fibre may lead to many disorders of the bowel, from constipation to cancer.

There are two types of dietary fibre: rapidly fermented (soluble) and slowly fermented (insoluble). Soluble fibre is found mostly in fruits, oats, barley and legumes, and insoluble fibre mainly in vegetables and grains. Both types of fibre assist the body in different ways.

Adequate fibre ensures that you stay regular. Foods containing fibre bind to water and help drag digested foods through your intestines. This ensures that food you eat passes through your body quite quickly after digestion. The last thing you want or need is to have a lot of toxic material hanging around in your body.

The benefits of fibre include an efficient and healthy digestive system, and feeling lighter and better. The most important reason to consume dietary fibre is to reduce your risk of colon cancer, which is the third most common cancer in the world. The recommended daily intake of fibre is 30–50 grams per day, depending on your size.

Generally speaking, foods with a high fibre content and a low Glycemic Index are those in their most natural state. That is fruits, vegetables, grains, bran, wheat germ, beans and other legumes. Highly processed foods will generally have low fibre content and be high GI, and should be avoided.

Choose Wisely

While an understanding and awareness of GI is important, GI is not the only consideration.

Remember when low fat was the 'be all and end all' and every time we went shopping or eating all we cared about was whether the food was low fat? Well we know what happened as a consequence of that short sightedness. In addition to the fat content, we needed to consider the effect of sugars and highly refined carbohydrates.

The same awareness must apply when considering the GI of a food. Remember that just because a food has a low GI it doesn't necessarily mean that it can be eaten in large amounts or that it is even a healthy choice. You need to take into account many other factors about a food such as:

- Its state, natural or processed

- Fat content and type

- Caloric content and your levels of activity

- An understanding of all ingredients

- Artificial additives.

A little bit of knowledge can be dangerous. Make sure you fully understand all implications and effects of foods.

Summary

1   Aim to raise your blood sugar levels to an optimum level and then maintain those levels for the day, every day.

2   Being organised is the first step to achieving this. That means being prepared and having the right food with you, so that when it is time to eat you are not caught out. If this means going to the supermarket more than once a week then I strongly recommend you do it.

3   The next step is to have an understanding and awareness of Glycemic Index, or GI. That is carbohydrate-containing foods and their effect on your blood sugar levels.

4   The combination of certain foods (protein, good fats and other low GI ingredients) will ensure a GI that is suitable for the type of meal.

5   By eating low GI meals on a regular and consistent basis you will be able to maintain a stable blood sugar level.

6   Eat fresh and natural foods, ie those high in nutrients, low GI and high in dietary fibre.

In the next chapter I will be talking specifically and practically about achieving your blood sugar objective. Before continuing, spend some time perusing the comprehensive list of the GI value of foods in the Appendix.

Supporting References

Savige, Dr G. et al., *Agefit* (2001), Pan Macmillan Australia.

Brand-Miller, J., *The New Glucose Revolution* (2002), Hodder Headline Australia Pty Ltd.

4
Achieving the Blood Sugar Objective

You have developed a relatively sound base of understanding to this point. I hope! Now we need to see how this can be applied into our real world and how simple it can be to make some minor changes to your eating to reap incredible rewards.

Case Study: Jane (Part 1)

I would like to introduce you to one of my clients. In the interest of privacy we will call her GI Jane.

When I first met Jane she was 40 years old, working three full days per week as a dental receptionist, mothering two children aged nine and 14, and training three mornings per week at the local gym.

Jane had been trying to lose fat for 14 years. Like so many people she had been on the diet and exercise round-about for that period of time. She had lost weight and put it back on so many times that she had almost lost the belief that she could look and feel the way she wanted to, and maintain it.

Her history was classic. Always quite lean and fit until after the birth of her first child, Jane became consumed with raising a new child, looking after a husband who was a workaholic, and going back to work within a relatively short period of time. Looking after herself slid very quickly to the bottom of the list.

High stress, a demanding family life and work commitments lead to inconsistent and emotional comfort eating and, consequently, Jane found herself:

- Overweight

- Lacking energy

- Emotional

- Out of control with food choices

- Inconsistent with exercise

- Not enjoying life.

It was at this point Jane was referred to me. A typical day for her was:

6am	out of bed
6–8am	organising, feeding and despatching husband and children
8am	cup of coffee, two pieces of white toast with butter and Vegemite or jam
9am	start work
10:30am	cup of coffee
1pm	chicken and salad sandwich, or a cup of soup with bread, or sushi
4pm	home from work with intense sugar cravings for lollies, chocolate, rice crackers, cake
4–6:30pm	preparing food, organising kids
7:30pm	dinner – pasta, stir fry and rice, roast and potatoes, pumpkin
9pm	sit down with a bowl of low fat ice cream, exhausted

On a day when she wasn't working, her time was filled with other chores and running around and so her eating regime was similar.

The first step was to give Jane an understanding of the things I have already discussed to this point. The next important understanding Jane needed was why she felt the way she did, and why it was so difficult for her to lose fat.

So, let's look at Jane's day a little closer:

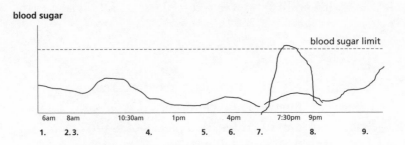

Graph 6 The effect of GI levels on blood sugar

Let me try to describe the graph in more detail:

1   When Jane gets up, her blood sugar levels are low. Since her last meal, her body has digested, processed and stored the majority of the food eaten, and her blood sugar levels have dropped to a low level.

2   From 6am to 8am Jane is out of bed and quite active in her duties. This requires energy so consequently her blood sugars will fall.

3   Her first meal is at 8am. She eats two pieces of white bread with butter and Vegemite or jam. The white bread has a high GI, but the butter and the jam or Vegemite will reduce the overall GI of the meal to one that is moderate. In addition the caffeine will cause a mild insulin response, further inhibiting a blood sugar increase.

4   By the time Jane gets to 10:30am her blood sugar levels have again begun to fall. The coffee at this time will only compound this drop.

5   By 1pm, a further 2½ hours later, and five hours after her last food intake her blood sugar levels are running on empty. Her lunch will again be one that is low to moderate in its GI, due to the combination of ingredients. This will cause a gradual rise in blood sugar levels, but still nowhere near its optimum.

6   A further three hours passes until the end of work or a chance to sit down briefly. It is at this point that Jane feels like that she has been hit by a bus and has an uncontrollable craving for something to give her an instant energy hit. Until this point her low blood sugar levels have affected Jane's day, but because her time has been so occupied she hasn't really noticed it. Now the mid-afternoon gremlins have got her!

7   In the afternoon, Jane would pretty much eat anything she could get her hands on. The effect on blood sugar levels will vary depending on what she eats. If she eats high GI food like lollies or rice crackers her blood sugar levels will rocket and then plummet (as illustrated in the graph). If she eats chocolate or cake or other high fat food, then the effect on her blood sugar levels will be far less extreme, due to the amount of fat the food contains (this is the lower line from 5 to 9pm in the graph).

8   Either way, by the time she gets to 7:30pm, her blood sugar levels are low again. Consequently dinner is likely to be a

much larger meal than she needs at this time of the day. A meal with large amounts of calories that her body must deal with in some way.

9   The need for ice cream at 9pm is again Jane's body craving sugar, as a hangover from a day lacking in calories and energy input and high in energy expenditure.

The effect of this type of eating on Jane's body is considerable. From the moment Jane gets out of bed at 6am she is active. This continues until she has finished cleaning up after dinner at about 8:30pm. That's 14½ hours!

During the period of the day from 6am to 4pm, when she needs optimal energy, she eats two pieces of toast and sometimes just a cup of soup! Her body is craving energy. It is in this situation, over a period of time, that her body will start to store body fat and break down lean muscle for energy. The consequent slowing effect on her metabolism means that the uncontrollable eating that begins at 4pm and continues through until 9:30pm is devastating. Her body has to deal with the large amounts of food consumed in this time. There is limited space in the already depleted muscle, which can only leave the fat cells as a viable storage site to accept the excess. All signs point to rapidly increasing fat levels and continually low energy levels.

Psychologically, the effects are just as damaging. Increasing levels of body fat decrease Jane's self image and consequently her self esteem. Her lack of energy and consequent reduced ability to perform daily functions (including work, home duties and training) create frustration and further doubts in her self worth. The uncontrollable cravings in the latter part of the day compound her beliefs that she has no willpower and will never be able to achieve her ideal situation.

So, Jane had developed a very negative pattern of behaviour for herself. One that she felt helpless to escape, but would have to change if she was to move forward.

The first thing Jane needed to realise was that positive change wouldn't require an extreme or unrealistic effort. She had always thought that to get any reasonable results she had to exercise for hours on end and considerably restrict her calorie intake. I was about to send her head into a bit of a spin.

The most important thing that I can say is that long-term change takes time and consistency. It requires choosing maybe one or two crucial areas (out of possibly 50) to start with, and putting time and effort into changing those particular behaviours. Once they are under control, it is about choosing a couple more aspects to focus on. Over time (maybe one to two years if necessary) the whole list will be attended to and those 'unattainable' goals will be achieved. The most important thing is that it must be gradual, realistic, enjoyable and fit in with an already established lifestyle.

In Jane's situation, we had to make only a few minor changes. To a certain extent, the rest would take care of itself.

Jane's day begins at 6am, so that is exactly when her eating should begin.

We know that when Jane gets up her blood sugar levels will be well down, so she needs to eat something that will raise these levels rapidly. This is one of those times when a high GI food is the best choice. Jane, like most people, found it hard to eat straight out of bed. My suggestion was something easy to eat and natural like a small amount of fruit: watermelon, cantaloupe or pineapple. These fruits are easy to prepare, easy to eat, fresh and natural and have a high GI. Jane decided she could handle a slice of watermelon at just after 6am.

The aim of this first meal is to get Jane's blood sugars up towards that optimal level. However, if Jane limited her initial food intake to this small amount of high GI fruit then her blood sugar levels would fall just as rapidly as they rose.

The next step is a crucial one in terms of the timing. Within 15 to 20 minutes, but no more than 30 minutes after the first high GI food intake, a second low GI meal is imperative. This meal is to stop the blood sugars from rising too high and to stabilise them around the optimal level. For most people this meal would be breakfast, but Jane felt she was unable to sit down to a proper breakfast until her family had been organised and despatched – we had to buy some time. I suggested a piece of low GI fruit, like an apple, pear or mandarin to keep her blood sugar levels from dropping and maintain them until breakfast could be eaten. She felt she could handle this.

At 8am it was breakfast time. Jane's meal had to again be low GI, as does every meal from this point, to maintain her blood sugar at the ideal level. We had to make a few minor, yet significant, changes to this meal. Instead of white bread we had to look for a more natural, lower GI substitute such as soy and linseed, sourdough rye, 100 percent rye or multi-grain. We were able to agree to either reduce the amount of butter or margarine or substitute it with avocado (a healthy fat that would help to reduce GI). She agreed on an all natural, sugar free jam and we discussed some other GI lowering ideas for her toast such as low fat cottage cheese, tomato or egg (occasionally).

Jane didn't feel like she could give up her breakfast coffee, so we decided she could keep having that one. I just reinforced with her that it was important to eat some food with the coffee to compensate for the insulin response and blood sugar drop the caffeine could cause.

At 10:30am it is time to eat again. Any more than 2½ to three hours and blood sugar levels are going to start falling. This meal needed to be a simple, convenient and low GI one to fit in with Jane's day. We decided that she felt comfortable eating an apple, a nectarine, a mandarin or some yoghurt at this time. Just enough to keep her blood sugar and hence energy levels sustained until lunch.

Her lunch at 1pm didn't really need to change. The chicken and salad sandwich was fine if Jane used a more wholegrain low GI bread (as above) and avocado instead of butter or margarine. Soup with low GI bread was a good option as long as the soup included protein, fresh and natural low GI ingredients and was low in saturated and synthetic fats. Sushi as an occasional meal is fine. Even though the rice is likely to be very high GI the raw fish will reduce its effect on blood sugar levels.

So far Jane would have eaten five times, so by the time the usual mid-afternoon cravings hit, she should be in total control. Her blood sugar levels maintained for the day meant that when it came to 3:30–4pm she was able to choose a snack that would take the edge off her hunger until dinnertime. We decided that her afternoon snack options would include fruit as earlier, yoghurt or a few almonds and dried apricots. Depending on the time of dinner I suggested another snack may be appropriate.

I highly recommended that Jane significantly reduce the size of her dinner. This is something that could only be done if enough of the right sort of food had been eaten regularly during the day. To eat a small dinner when food intake during the day has been minimal and blood sugar levels are low is like a 'lead foot' trying to drive a red convertible turbo Porsche on an open road on a sunny day and keeping it under 10 kph. It won't happen!

It really is crucial at this time of the day, when Jane's energy expenditure is reduced, to keep caloric intake to a minimum. Any excess calories the body can't deal with either by storing as energy in the muscle or using quite readily will be stored in the only place left – FAT CELLS!

Any evening meal with large amounts of high calorie foods such as pasta, rice, bread, potatoes and pumpkin should be reduced. This rocked Jane's world at first. The thought of reducing the staple of her evening meal seemed incomprehensible. 'What am I supposed to eat?' she pleaded.

It wasn't that difficult to let her see the myriad options available. Stir fry's with lean meat and vegetables, grilled fish and green vegetables, omelettes, casseroles and curries, roasted meats with low GI vegetables. The difference between these meals and what she was used to was the size of the serve and the reduced amount of pasta, rice, bread, potatoes, pumpkin, etc.

After dinner the assumption is that Jane has eaten enough food throughout the day and really doesn't need to eat any more. In addition, any craving that she would normally have should no longer exist due to her newly controlled blood sugar levels. The occasional after dinner snack or dessert is encouraged, as long as the decision is based on choice not compulsion.

Jane's new eating plan looked something like this:

6am	out of bed
6:05am	small amount of watermelon
6:25am	one apple, pear or orange
8am	cup of coffee, two pieces of soy and linseed toast with avocado, tomato, low fat cottage cheese and/or jam (no added sugar)
10:30am	a piece of low GI fruit (apple, pear or mandarin) and/or some yoghurt
1pm	chicken, turkey or tuna and salad in soy and linseed sandwich, or home made soup with lots of vegetables, beans, lentils and some protein with approved bread, or sushi (occasionally)
4pm	yoghurt, almonds and/or dried apricots
7pm	dinner – a small serve of chicken and vegetable stir fry, fish and salad with only a small amount of basmati rice, sweet potato or noodles, if any
9pm	an occasional snack or treat (one or two times per week)

Implementation of Your Objectives

The next step is to implement this plan into your life with minimal disruption and maximum effect. Here are some things to consider:

- If you can't do it all at once, that's okay!

- Choose the most crucial aspects of your eating and start with those. For example, if you don't eat breakfast you will reap a huge benefit if the only change you make is to eat something as soon as you get up. Once the breakfast routine is established, move to the next.

- Most people find that the morning routine is the one that will have the greatest bearing on their day, so that is where I suggest you begin.

- Initially aim to follow the plan quite closely from Monday to Friday and allow yourself some indulgence on the weekend. Weekdays seem to be easier to establish routine.

- Be organised with your food:
    (i)   Go shopping and stock the shelves and fridge at home and work with the right stuff.
    (ii) Pre-prepare food when you have the time and package it, freezing it if necessary, so you have great meals ready to go.
    (iii) Have a survival kit of food with you at all times so that you are never caught out without food, or with less than ideal options (see snack options later).

- In the early stages you may need to remind yourself to eat, until your body starts to remind you. Set an alarm clock, leave yourself notes, use your computer or get someone else to remind you when it is time to eat.

- Experiment with different foods until you find meals you really enjoy and which control your blood sugar levels. I have included a list of suggested foods and ingredients for each meal towards the end of this chapter.

- Don't count calories and don't measure food – all this will do is make your life difficult and promote obsessive behaviour patterns.

- Eat enough so that you are satisfied, but not over-full, and don't leave yourself hungry. If you are still hungry there is a greater likelihood that you will overeat at the end of the day.

- If you are unsure whether you are satisfied, wait 20 minutes. This is the time it takes the message that you are full to get from your stomach to your brain. Often, even if you still feel hungry straight after eating, you won't 20 minutes later.

- Watch for signs of low blood sugar levels, e.g. cravings, lethargy, moodiness.

- Low blood sugar is usually because:
    (i) You have not had your high GI fruit as soon as getting up.
    (ii) You've gone more than three hours without eating.
    (iii) You have eaten a high GI food at some stage during the day without following it up with a low GI food within 15–20 minutes.
    (iv) You have drunk too much caffeine.

If for one of the above reasons you allow your blood sugar level to drop, get it back to where you want it by eating a high GI food followed by a low GI food within 15–20 minutes.

- Set yourself progressive goals in certain areas. For example if you drink five cups of coffee per day and your ideal goal is two per day, take it gradually. That is, in the first week aim for four cups per day – still too many, but at least it is better. The next week or two aim for three. Over a period of maybe four to eight weeks you may have achieved your ideal two cups per day.

- If you try to change too much too quickly, chances are that it won't last and you will end up back where you started.

- Always think LIFETIME. If you can't maintain it long term, then don't even try.

- Make sure you allow yourself some indulgences. We all know that alcohol, chocolate and take-away food are not ideal in terms of health. However, if you really enjoy them then allow yourself the occasional treat. DO NOT feel guilty – in the 'big picture' the small amount we are talking about will have a negligible negative effect on your body. The effect they will have on your enjoyment of eating and balance of living far outweighs any physical consequence. I will discuss this in more depth in Chapter 11.

Eating Options

The great thing about this way of eating is that the food options available to you are enormous. Jane's eating plan is just one that suited her. If you can just remember a few golden rules then you can write your own plan with all the foods you enjoy.

The Golden Rules of Food Choices

1 Choose foods that are generally low in saturated fats (i.e. animal fats and vegetable oils) and trans-fatty acids (i.e. synthetic fats in processed, snack and take-away foods).

2 Don't be afraid of foods with good fats, e.g. olive, canola and flaxseed oil, avocado, almonds, fish in moderation.

3 Choose foods that have no or minimal added sugars.

4 Avoid highly processed and refined foods.

5 Choose fresh, natural and wholegrain foods.

6 Eat heaps of fruit and vegetables.

7 Be aware of the GI of the foods you buy.

8 Think about the combination of foods you will be eating and their effect on overall GI.

9 Choose foods you enjoy.

The High GI Options

These are for first thing in the morning and/or straight after cardio training (see Chapter 10):

Fruit
Watermelon, canteloupe, honeydew melon and pineapple.

Juices
Made with the above listed fruits.

Sports Drinks
To have after exercise.

Breakfast Options (low GI)

Cereals, Oats and Natural Muesli
See the GI list in the Appendix and choose the most natural and low to moderate options. Some healthy and yummy additions to cereal include:

- Low fat milk

- Yoghurt – preferably natural, low fat with no added sugar

- Low or moderate GI fruit (berries, kiwi, grapes, apple, pear, peach) – fresh or stewed

- Flaxseed oil (a great source of omega 3 fat)

- LSA (linseed, sunflower seeds and almonds)

- Yellow box or other low GI honey.

Make a smoothie with cereals and any or all of the above ingredients.

Toast

Preferably soy and linseed, 100 percent rye, sourdough rye or grainy bread, with any combination of the following:

- Spreads – Yellow box honey, Vegemite, jam (no added sugar), avocado (instead of butter/margarine), peanut or almond butter (in moderation)

- Low fat cottage or ricotta cheese (in moderation)

- Eggs – poached, boiled or microwaved (use at least one yolk, but no more than two)

- Lean ham, bacon, chicken, tuna

- Tomato, spinach, mushrooms

Snack Options (low GI)

Quick and Easy

These are for the survival kit (to go):

- Fresh low GI fruit

- Fruit cups/packs (no added sugar)

- Yoghurt

- Nuts (almonds, macadamias and walnuts), seeds and dried fruit (apple, apricot, prunes and other low- to moderate-GI fruits)

- Protein shake

- Some bars (see Chapter 8 for more info)

- Vitaweat biscuits with spreads (as above)

- Left-overs from the night before

Snacks Which Require Some Preparation

- Smoothies or juices

- Soups

- Toast (as breakfast)

- Sandwich (see lunch options)

- Vitaweat biscuits with cottage cheese and tomato, avocado and chicken

- Left-overs that require heating.

Lunch Options (low GI)

Sandwiches, Rolls or Wraps

With approved low to moderate GI bread. Fillers:

- Lean protein – chicken, ham, meat, tuna, salmon, egg, low fat cheese

- Salad stuff (as you like)

- Spreads and condiments – avocado, mustards (watch sugar content), hommus, tahini, almond butter.

Rice Dishes

Use brown long grain, long grain, basmati or Doongara. Include:

- Some protein (chicken, tuna, lean meat, eggs, tofu, beans, lentils)

- Low GI vegetable (broccoli, cauliflower, capsicum, onion, mushroom, zucchini, beans, tomato, peas)

- Herbs, spices and flavours (watch fat and sugar content)

Examples: curries, casseroles, stir fries, sushi and Californian rolls.

Soups
Use low GI ingredients, low saturated fat and no added sugar.

- Sweet potato

- Lentil

- Vegetable

- Minestrone

- Chicken and vegetable

- Pea and ham.

Include some low GI bread or rice and some form of protein if needed.

Salads

- Tuna, chicken, lamb, beef, calamari, octopus, tofu, egg

- Sweet potato, beans, bread

- If dressing is required include olive oil, balsamic vinegar, lemon juice etc.

Pasta

Use fresh or fast-cooking pasta.

• Ideally with a tomato base

• Include some quality protein and fresh vegetables.

Pasta should be an occasional meal. While pasta is relatively low GI, it takes effort and energy to digest, which may have an impact on your energy levels.

Afternoon Snack Options (low GI)

As for morning snack options (see page 67).

Dinner Options

Dinner should be a small meal.

Protein
Chicken, turkey, fish, lean red meat, egg, tofu, lentils, beans, chickpeas etc.

Low GI Vegetables or Salad Stuff
At this time of the day, limit the amount of rice, pasta, potatoes, sweet potatoes, bread, cereals and other starches (regardless of GI). Examples:

• Stir fries

• Casseroles and curries

• Meat/chicken/fish and salad or vegies

• Omelettes

• BBQs and salad.

For more ideas see our recipe section, Part Two.

Recommended Eating Guidelines

To give you more ideas how to structure your eating have a look at the following general guidelines. Use the guidelines as an ultimate eating plan, i.e. something to work toward. Pick one, two or as many areas to concentrate on as you can, at one time. Once they have been established as routines, choose one or some more. Obviously, the closer you can follow these guidelines the better. BUT remember we are interested in long term results, so if it takes some time to get your eating right in the long term then you have been successful.

1   Eat a **small amount of high GI fruit** as soon as getting up. For example; watermelon, cantaloupe, honeydew melon or pineapple.

2   Eat breakfast **15–20 minutes** later. Breakfast options include:
    - Oats, natural muesli, wholegrain cereal with natural low-fat yoghurt and/or low GI fruit (e.g. apple, pear or mandarin).
    - Toast (100 percent rye, sourdough rye, soy and linseed or other wholegrain bread) with naturally sweetened jam, Vegemite or similar product, tomato. Include either low fat cottage cheese, eggs (one yolk only) or lean ham or chicken. Use minimal butter or margarine; substitute with avocado.

3   Snack **every two hours** until lunch – low GI fruit, low fat yoghurt, almonds and dried apricots, protein shake, Vitaweat biscuits with toppings (as for breakfast).

4   **Lunch**

    Lunch options include:
    - Sandwich, roll or wrap (soy and linseed, 100 percent rye, sourdough rye, rye mountain bread) with lean meat, chicken, turkey, tuna, egg etc

and salad. NO butter, marg or mayo – use avocado.

- Basmati rice with lean protein (as above) and vegetables. NOT fried in oil.
- Sweet potato with the above.
- Occasionally pasta with a tomato base, lean protein and vegetables. NO oil.

5 **Mid-afternoon snack** (every two hours; one or two depending on the time between lunch and dinner). Food options same as morning snack.

6 Eat **dinner as early as possible** for you. It should consist of fish, lean chicken or red meat (or other protein) with low GI salad or vegetables.
- **Reduce the amount** of pasta, rice, bread, potatoes etc., with a view to eliminating them.
- **Avoid eating after dinner,** except for occasional indulgences. Generally, if you are still hungry, you need to increase your food intake during the day.
- Allow yourself the occasional indulgence.
- Drink **at least two to three litres of water** each day (not including water consumed during exercise).
- Limit **caffeine intake to two cups** of tea or coffee (with meals) per day. Use herbal tea as a preference.
- Be very aware of the **negative effect alcohol** has on your body and consume accordingly.
- **Recommended spreads, sauces and flavours** – Vegemite or similar product, naturally sweetened jam, almond spread or peanut butter (in moderation), sugar-free soy/tamari, lemon juice, mustard, naturally sweetened chutney, red wine, curry powder, tomato paste (no added sugar), herbs and spices.

Food Diary

I recommend that you start keeping a food diary. If you are really serious about creating long-term change then this is a vital tool.

What is a food diary and why keep one? Good questions!

A food diary is a journal of your eating, drinking, moods and energy levels. Each day you record everything that goes into your mouth, including times and approximate amounts (no need to be ridiculously accurate). Each day you make some note of your mood and energy levels at different stages during the day. The aim is to create awareness and under-standing about the relationship between the way you feel and the way you are eating.

If you are tired, lethargic, cranky and craving sugar then chances are that you have let your blood sugar levels drop throughout the day. If you have kept an accurate food diary you will be able to identify how and when it happened.

On the other hand if you feel fantastic and have a consis-tently high energy level then it is important to be able to see what and how you have eaten during that day to ensure that this day can be repeated.

If you understand how eating a certain way will make you feel then you are more likely to change or keep going as the case dictates. The food diary need only be kept for a rela-tively short time (two to six months) until this awareness and understanding is established.

For a Sample Food Diary, please see page 401.

Case Study: Jane (Part 2)

After all that, you are probably wondering what happened to Jane! Well you will be happy to know that it is a happy ending so far. I have been working with Jane for about three years. The first 12 months were the greatest challenge for her as she tried to change habits, beliefs and attitudes that she had lived by up to that time.

The first thing she began to notice was that she had more energy; she was more productive and more motivated to exercise. There were times when she slipped up, but over time I helped her to understand that as long she got back on track and didn't beat herself up over it, then this occasional slip-up was harmless and, in fact, necessary. She needed to understand that no one is perfect and everyone needs to indulge occasionally.

In the three years since Jane and I have been associated she has achieved the following:

- She has lost about 10kg (22lb) of fat, and with the exception of one or two kg variation, has kept it off.

- She is still losing fat.

- She has kept an accurate and honest food diary, which I have checked every week, and we have gradually fine-tuned her eating to a point where she can now happily maintain it forever.

- Her eating plan includes alcohol and chocolate in moderate amounts.

- She ran a half marathon (21km) last year, having never run more than 5km in her life.

- She is lifting weights that she never thought she could lift.

- She has a job in an advertising agency, three days a week, and is achieving great things.

- She has convinced her husband to follow a similar plan and they now have much more in common (he has lost 8kg so far) and they have the time and energy to spend quality time with their children and each other.

- She is happy and knows that this way of life for her and her family will last forever.

Well done, Jane, you are a champion.

5
Facts on Fats

I have gone a fair way into this book without discussing fat in a lot of detail. I thought I would keep you in suspense for as long as possible! Now is the time to bring out the big guns!

Don't worry, there is no need to be scared. Although I know most people are terrified of this four-letter word – F A T S!

There is a huge amount of misinformation about fats. As a result of this misleading information we have largely correlated **all** dietary fat with that same horrible stuff that sits on our stomachs and hips or in our arteries contributing to heart disease. To compound the problem, very few people in positions of authority have made any effort to tell us anything to the contrary. In fact many health professionals continue to condemn all fats as the enemy. No wonder we have become so fat phobic!

The fact is, an outer covering called a cell membrane encloses every cell in our body. This membrane is made up of 75 percent fat consisting of healthy, natural fats including essential fatty acids Omega 3 and Omega 6, some saturated fats and cholesterol. A healthy cell membrane will easily allow nutrients to enter and nourish the cell. The consumption of too little fat or the wrong type of fat will compromise the membrane and its ability to allow nutrients to enter.

The Four Fats

There are four types of fats. Some foods contain a combination of polyunsaturated and monounsaturated fats and are therefore included in more than one list.

- Saturated – animal fats, milk products and coconut oil

- Polyunsaturated
    (i) Omega 3 – fish (salmon, tuna, mackerel, sardines, trevally, trout), flaxseed oil, walnuts, almonds, pumpkin seeds and linseeds, Omega 3-enriched eggs
    (ii) Omega 6 – usually from vegetable oils, leafy vegetables, grains, seeds, nuts, lean meat and chicken

- Monounsaturated – olive oil, avocado and nuts (almonds, walnuts and macadamias)

- Trans-Fatty Acids – processed and fast foods, including those advertised as low in fat (for example margarine, doughnuts, muffins, rice crackers, breakfast bars and many other convenience, processed and take-away foods).

All the above fats, with the exception of one, are naturally occurring. Trans-fatty acids are a synthetic or processed form of unsaturated fats that occur when healthy fats, which are liquid at room temperature, are converted to a solid by a process called chemical hydrogenation.

This chemical process is used commercially to make the fat easier and cheaper to use on a large scale and to last longer. It allows products to be advertised as containing healthy unsaturated fats – many with no mention of the new and potentially harmful fat that has resulted. This synthetic fat should be consumed with caution and in moderation.

Saturated Fats

Saturated fats tend to get a worse rap than they deserve. Yes, we should aim to reduce saturated fats as, according to Dr Ross Walker, cardiologist, it is estimated that a 5 percent increase in saturated fat consumption will contribute to a 17 percent increase in risk of heart disease. However, some lean meat or chicken, in moderation, contributes to a healthy and well-balanced eating plan and plays a crucial role in the make-up of a healthy cell membrane.

Polyunsaturated and Monounsaturated Fats

These are **good fats** that will contribute to the prevention of disease and the maintenance of a healthy body.

Monounsaturated fats have been shown to lower LDL (bad) cholesterol and possibly raise HDL (good) cholesterol (see later in this chapter for more on cholesterol). They decrease blood clotting (a contributor to stroke, deep vein thrombosis and heart disease) and may reduce hypertension.

Polyunsaturated fats include Omega 3 and Omega 6 fats. These are referred to as **essential fatty acids** (EFA) as they are essential to a healthy existence but cannot be produced by the body. They therefore must be supplied via food.

Essential fatty acids improve heart health by reducing bad LDL blood cholesterol, blood pressure and blood clotting. These fatty acids are also needed for brain development in infants. EFA reduces inflammation in people with arthritis and may help reduce the severity of mental and behavioural disorders.

In Australia we eat Omega 6 and Omega 3 fats in a ratio of about 10:1. A ratio of 3:1 is a far healthier target and means we need to decrease our consumption of Omega 6 fats and increase Omega 3 sources. I would highly recommend a quality Omega 3 supplement for anyone lacking in this crucial nutrient.

Trans-Fatty Acids

Trans-fatty acids contribute to the majority of health concerns of the modern time. Dr Walker has revealed that some studies even show that a 2 percent increase in the consumption of trans-fatty acids can increase cardiac risk by up to 93 percent! This means that even foods advertised as low fat would cause serious health problems if the small amount of fat were primarily made up of trans-fatty acids, as most of them are. The major concern is that in this time of high convenience and processed foods, our unconscious consumption of these trans-fatty acids is increasing.

The potential problem occurs at the cellular level. The cell membrane has trouble distinguishing between natural occurring fats and synthetic or processed fats in the form of trans-fatty acids. When these trans-fatty acids are introduced into the body they become a part of the cell membrane, rearranging it and making it hard and impenetrable to nutrients. These nutrients include fats, carbohydrates (in the form of glucose) and proteins. They also include vitamins and minerals. So you can understand the drastic effect this must create when the body is deprived of all these vital nutrients.

Remember our goal is to live an **energised, lean and healthy life**? It may be severely compromised by consuming trans-fatty acids. The malnourished cells will lack the nutrients they need to effectively perform their tasks. They will lack energy and consequently this will contribute to any feelings of lethargy that you may experience. **You will have less energy.**

If the cell membrane is unable to allow vital nutrients to pass through, think of the consequences. For example consider sugar. In Chapter 3 I spoke about insulin's role of transporting sugar to the muscle and liver cells for storage and use. I also mentioned insulin as being responsible for storing any excess sugar as fat. The altered cell state, due to trans-fatty acid consumption, makes it difficult for insulin to transport the sugar across the hard cell membrane, thus leaving excess in the blood. Consequently the body produces even more insulin to cope with this excess. As the body becomes more resistant to this insulin, due to the cells' deformed membranes, more insulin will be produced. A high level of insulin in the blood will result in the excess sugar being stored as fat. **We will get fatter.**

Continual and excessive production of insulin puts enormous strain on the pancreas. Over a long period of time this can quite possibly lead to pancreas damage. This damage affects the pancreas' ability to produce insulin and hence the body's ability to control the level of sugar in the blood. This may lead to a condition known as **type II diabetes**, one of the most prevalent diseases of modern time.

Cholesterol

'Aaagh, cholesterol! I'm really not that sure what it is or does, all I know is that it is dangerous. Keep it away from me!' This is a common attitude towards cholesterol that I experience from many of my clients.

Cholesterol has got a much worse rap than it deserves, simply because many people don't understand it. I am not going to get too scientific here, but I do want to clarify some important points – to give you the full story.

Okay, so what is it? Well I will tell you what it isn't – fat! Yes, you read correctly. It is actually a pearly coloured, waxy-type substance that is crucial in many ways. Where would we find it? Most people would suggest in the bloodstream where it can cause its damage. In fact Dr Michael Eales, M.D., in his book *Protein Power* suggests that only 7 percent of cholesterol is found in the blood, while 93 percent contributes to the make up of cell membranes. Its waxy nature allows the regulation of nutrients and waste products entering and leaving cells.

What I am saying is that cholesterol is far from the villain it is made out to be. In fact it is critical to human life. If you still don't believe me, have a look at some of the other benefits of cholesterol.

- Cholesterol is the building block from which your body makes important hormones.

- Cholesterol aids in the digestion of foods, especially fatty foods.

- Cholesterol is needed for brain and nerve development.

- Cholesterol allows the skin to shed water.

- Cholesterol helps the body convert sunlight to vitamin D.

- Cholesterol is needed for tissue growth and repair.

- Cholesterol helps transport blood fats through the body.

Not such a bad thing after all!

However, cholesterol becomes a problem when consumed in excess, as it elevates blood cholesterol. Cholesterol in the cell membrane can be regulated; in the blood it cannot. Therefore excess blood cholesterol will be stored in the lining of the artery walls, hence the negative effect that we are well aware of.

You may have heard that total blood cholesterol is made from two types of cholesterol: high density lipoprotein or HDL (good), and low density lipoprotein or LDL (bad). Cholesterol is not soluble in the blood, so for it to be transported through the blood it must be enclosed in a blood-soluble envelope called lipoprotein.

LDL cholesterol is the villain because it attaches itself to the artery walls where blockages can occur. HDL cholesterol comes to the rescue because it travels through the blood collecting LDL cholesterol from the arteries and then transporting it to the liver for recycling or removal from the body.

The goal is to therefore increase HDL and reduce LDL cholesterol. Here are some tips:

1 Reduce your consumption of take-away foods and highly processed fats, carbohydrates and sugars.

2 Increase your intake of monounsaturated and polyunsaturated fats from natural sources.

3 Eat mainly natural foods, which have a low GI, to ensure your blood sugar levels don't rise too rapidly. Excess insulin will activate the enzyme that fuels cholesterol production. Excess insulin may also contribute to smooth muscle growth on the artery wall, increasing blood pressure.

4 Dr Ross Walker in *The Cell Factor* suggests that stress and metabolism can have varying effects on cholesterol production. Deal with any stress you may have and ensure your metabolism is functioning as effectively as possible through healthy eating and regular exercise.

Summary

1 Don't be fat phobic.

2 Include some healthy monounsaturated and polyunsaturated fats in your plan.

3 Enjoy some natural and lean meat and chicken in moderation.

4 Avoid highly processed foods and trans-fatty acids.

Supporting References

Walker, Dr R., *The Cell Factor* (2002), Pan Macmillan Australia.

Eades, Dr Michael & Dr Mary, *Protein Power* (1999), Bantam Books.

6

The Power of Protein

I have talked about carbohydrates at length and their vital importance in your eating plan. I have explained the importance of fat for your body, and how we need not be so fat phobic! Now it is time to discuss the third crucial piece of the nutrient puzzle – protein.

Like fats and carbohydrates I'm sure you have heard a lot about protein, good and bad, accurate or inaccurate. A portion of the population swear by protein because they think the more they eat the bigger muscles they will get, and so they consume copious amounts of egg whites, chicken fillets, steaks, tuna, protein bars and gallons of protein shakes. Another segment of the population will steer away from protein, particularly animal protein because of the perceived fat content or because they are vegetarian, and so they risk not fulfilling their protein needs.

Protein, as with carbohydrates and fats, is a vital nutrient for the efficient functioning of the body. It must be consumed in sufficient quantities without being over-consumed as occurs in many cases.

Protein helps to build, maintain and repair almost every part of our bodies. The quality of your hair, nails, skin, cartilages, tendons and muscles is largely determined by the quality of your protein. In addition to growth and repair, it is important in the production of enzymes (compounds made from protein that speed up the chemical reactions in the body), antibodies, hormones and other important body components.

There are two common misconceptions about protein:

1 The more you eat, the bigger your muscles will be.

2 The only quality protein comes from animals.

Firstly, your body can handle only so much protein. If you consume too much, then as with any excess, your body will store it as fat. In addition to this fat storage, an over-abundance of protein can potentially create serious kidney and liver damage and disease. The recommended daily intake is suggested below. But as with all recommended intakes, it doesn't take into account individual differences. If you're unsure, seek professional advice.

As for the second myth – that the only quality protein comes from animals – well, a more inaccurate statement has never been made. I will explore this further as we progress.

Recommended Daily Intake (RDI) of Protein

Sedentary person	0.75g per kg body weight per day
Moderately exercising person	0.9–1.2g per kg body weight per day
Highly active person	1.2–1.7g per kg body weight per day

Protein is formed by building blocks called amino acids. There are approximately 22 different kinds of amino acids that form billions of combinations of proteins. Out of the 22 amino acids there are eight that our bodies do not manufacture. We must get these through the food we eat and they are referred to as essential amino acids.

These essential amino acids are called:

- Valine

- Leucine

- Isoleucine

- Lysine

- Tryptophan

- Methionine

- Phenylalanine

- Histidine.

I'm sure you will remember these and go around showing off by reciting them. Well maybe not! The myth that animal protein is the only source of quality protein comes from the misinformed opinion that only animal protein provides 'complete proteins'. A 'complete protein' is one that contains all eight of the essential amino acids.

Yes it is true that animal proteins are complete proteins, but it is also very true that the amino acids that come from plant foods are exactly the same as amino acids that come from animal foods.

Before we progress any further, let's have a look at the different sources of protein.

Animal Sources

- All animal meats – beef, lamb, pork, chicken, turkey, fish, seafood etc.

- Dairy products – milk, cheese, yoghurt, cream etc.

- Eggs – the white and a small amount of yolk must be present to form a complete protein. The minimum required ratio of yolk to white is 1:6.

Plant Sources

- Nuts and seeds

- Pulses/legumes – soy beans and soy products (e.g. tofu), beans, peas, chickpeas, lentils and split peas

- Grains – brown rice, wholegrain breads, wholegrain pasta

- Vegetables – sweetcorn, broccoli and carrots are the vegetables with the highest protein content

If you are a vegan or a vegetarian, then all is okay. You can quite easily give yourself sufficient, high-quality complete proteins. You just need to remember a basic rule in terms of combining your food to produce a complete protein. It is a simple matter of eating a **grain with a pulse, legume and/or nut**. And don't forget to include your other vegetables to complete the meal.

Here are some examples:

- Rice and beans

- Lentil soup with wholegrain bread

- Wholegrain pasta with a lentil or bean bolognaise

- Stir-fried tofu with vegetables and rice.

Protein Supplements

Clients often ask me about protein bars and protein powders.

Over the last five to 10 years, supplements have become more commonplace, readily available and accepted in many people's lives. Many people are driven by the thought that they can get the edge over the next person and will spend a significant amount of money on supplements. In the gym and personal training environment, it is hard to avoid the push to get onto the protein supplement train.

If you are deficient in your protein consumption, or if your protein requirements are increased, then the use of controlled protein supplementation can be quite beneficial. But I certainly wouldn't encourage you to use supplements in place of quality fresh and natural protein sources. Many people rely on bars and powders for the majority of their protein intake. Remember, they are a processed food and as such contain many artificial ingredients that may be harmful. However, in moderation and after advice from a trusted professional, then I say go for it.

Eat a Balance of Protein

Complete proteins are available from myriad sources. I recommend that you eat from as many of these sources as possible. Not only will this increase the variety of foods you eat and hence the enjoyment, it will also ensure that you gain all the associated health benefits.

Remember that protein included with your meals helps to maintain your blood sugar at the level required to contribute to ongoing energy.

Animal protein need not be avoided because of perceived fat storage. Simply trim all fat from your meat and cook it in such a way that excess fat drains off.

If you are a vegetarian, be clear about the foods you can eat and the combinations that will produce complete proteins. You need to be able to avoid animal products and still enjoy the benefits of quality protein. If you are unsure, seek help from a qualified dietician or nutritionist.

Supporting References

Savige, Dr G. et al., *Agefit* (2001), Pan Macmillan Australia.

Walker, Dr R., *The Cell Factor* (2002), Pan Macmillan Australia.

7
Water, Vitamins, Minerals and Phytochemicals – the Quiet Achievers

As I mentioned in Chapter 2, there are six nutrients that make up all food that we consume. The three less talked about but certainly no less important are water, vitamins and minerals. Other very useful chemicals found only in plants are called phytochemicals and whilst not considered essential are most certainly beneficial to optimal health.

Before I discuss these crucial nutrients I want you to understand exactly how important they are to your wellbeing and longevity.

Let me give you some statistics. (Keep in mind that these are relevant to the time of the research and are obviously subject to change, hopefully for the better.)

Did you know the following?

- **One in two** men and **one in three** women will develop coronary heart disease (1).

- Diabetes affects more than **430,000 Australians**. Estimates suggest that a further **350,000 are affected but unaware** (2). There are **250 new cases** of type II diabetes diagnosed each day (3).

- Even more recently it has been suggested that **1.2 million Australians** are diabetic and a further **two million are pre-diabetic** (that is, on the verge).

- Nearly **80,000 new cases** of cancer are diagnosed each year (4). It is estimated that **one in three** men and **one in four** women will be directly affected by cancer (5).

- **56 percent of Australians** are overweight or obese (6).

- Osteoporosis affects **one in two women** and **one in three men** over the age of 60 (7).

- Approximately **80 percent of these conditions** could be prevented by lifestyle changes: controlling stress, not smoking, having a good eating regime and taking regular exercise (8).

SOURCES

(1) 'Heart, Stroke and Vascular Disease: Australian Facts 1999', the Australian Institute of Health and Welfare and the Heart Foundation of Australia

(2) *Super Food Ideas* magazine, June/July 2000, p22

(3) *Australasian Doctor*, 20 October 2000, p41 'Exercise the best Strategy', The Australasian Society for the Study of Obesity – 9th Annual Scientific Meeting, Brisbane

(4) The National Cancer Statistics Clearing House of Australian Institute of Health and Welfare (AIHW).

(5) ABS statistics: data from the most up-to-date sources available, including data from the 1995 National Health Survey

(6) AIHW 1999, Heart, Stroke and Vascular Diseases: Australian Facts; AIHW Cat. No. CVD 7, Canberra: AIHW and the Heart Foundation of Australia (Cardiovascular Diseases Series No. 10)

(7) AFA – Osteoporosis Australia (data from Garvan Institute)

(8) *The Daily Telegraph* (3/7/00), p85 'Survival Instincts'

These are pretty alarming statistics, I think you will agree. The most alarming is that 80 percent of these life-threatening diseases and conditions are preventable!

It seems incredible that we hold the power to control the quality and length of our lives, yet many of us wait until our body starts to break down and then we pass responsibility to someone else to fix it.

By taking action now and making sure you are eating all the quality nutrients you need, you will save yourself lots of pain, heartache and money in the long run. Not to mention enjoying your life for many more years than your current lifestyle will allow.

Everything I have just said is not to scare you, but to emphasise the importance of a well-balanced eating plan, including all the crucial nutrients, in addition to carbo-hydrates, proteins and fats. But if it does scare you into action, then good!

Water

There is no resource more readily available, more vital to human life yet more taken for granted than water. Despite the incredible and immeasurable importance of water, do you truly realise and appreciate the significance of its role in your life?

There is not one bodily function that is not dependant on water. In fact, 70 percent of the body is water. Have a think about how your body would be without it – not much more than a pile of dust!

The following list gives the percentage of various body parts that are composed of water:

Teeth	10%
Bones	13%
Cartilage	55%
Red blood corpuscles	69%
Liver	72%
Muscle tissue	75%
Spleen	76%
Lungs	80%
Brain	81%
Bile	86%
Plasma	90%
Blood	91%
Lymph	94%
Gastric juice	96%
Saliva	96%

Is it time for a drink?!

Some of the more important functions of water are as follows:

1 Water supports and aids every bodily process from digestion and absorption of food and nutrients, to utilisation and excretion. From the moment food enters your mouth, every process to transform it from its original state to blood, bone, muscle and tissue relies on water.

2 As we know, food is broken down to the nutrients necessary for life through processes requiring water. Those nutrients are then held in solution and transported to the various body parts in water.

3 Water holds the wastes and toxins that it collects from the cells and carries them to the appropriate organs for elimination.

4 Water is a vital ingredient of all cells and tissues and of all body fluids. For example, saliva, gastric juices and blood are all over 90 percent water.

5 Water keeps various mucous membranes of the body soft and lubricated, and it prevents rubbing or friction between tissue surfaces. This enhances the body's ability to move, organs' abilities to function and the suppleness of muscles.

6 Water is the chief agent in regulating body temperature. This is vital, as an internal temperature change of only a few degrees can mean death.

Keeping all the above points in mind, you can imagine the dramatic effect of dehydration on the body. Most of the people I talk to suffer from mild to severe dehydration every day of their lives.

People who exercise are at an even higher risk as they will lose water through their body's cooling process. Dehydration can cause a decrease in physical performance, so whether you are competing in a sporting competition or trying to exercise regularly for fitness or fat loss benefits, dehydration will seriously hamper your progress.

This brings us to three questions that need to be answered. **When** should we drink water? **How much** water should we drink? **What** is the best type of water to drink?

When to Drink Water

When is an easy one. Your body will tell you when you need to drink, which is when you are thirsty. You need to be able to recognise the first indication of thirst as a warning that dehydration is imminent, and then act accordingly. Many people have taught themselves to ignore this feeling and may have desensitized themselves to the initial signs of thirst.

As a general rule, you should aim to drink a glass of water:

1 When you get up, before you eat or drink anything else

2 10 to 15 minutes before each meal

3 Any other time when thirst strikes.

Water may have a detrimental effect if consumed while you are eating or directly after eating. Because water leaves the stomach so quickly, it is fine to drink it before eating. Drinking water with or straight after a meal dilutes the gastric juices and carries them right out of the stomach. Drinking while eating may cause you to swallow only partially masticated food. Both of these situations will disrupt the digestive process and quite possibly lead to digestive complaints and stinky, antisocial behaviour!

Ideally, drinking should not happen during eating or within two hours of the completion of the meal. I understand, however, that practically this may be difficult to avoid consistently. I am suggesting that you are aware of the effects and take the necessary precautions whenever possible.

How Much Water Should I Drink?

When considering **how much** water to drink there are several things to take into account. The climate and activity levels will obviously affect the amount of water you need to consume. Thirst is very much related to the amount of water in the food that you eat. The less you get from food the more you need to drink. Eating a large amount of natural, unrefined foods, fruits and vegetables will provide you with more of your daily water requirements.

Try to be sensitive to your thirst and let your body tell you how much you need to drink. The colour of urine is another indicator of water balance. Clear urine suggests an adequate level of hydration; yellow and stinky urine is a sign that more water needs to be consumed.

There is no set amount that is appropriate for every person, so the old 'drink eight glasses a day' theory may be suitable for maybe 10 percent of the population. You need to work it out for yourself depending on your size, activity levels, the climate and the food that you eat.

An insufficient fluid intake can, in the short term, lead to headaches, constipation, fatigue, lack of appetite, light headedness and muscle cramps. Over the long term a lack of fluid increases the risk of kidney stones developing.

Many people ask me: 'Is it possible to drink too much water?' The answer is yes. A moderate excess of water will be passed relatively harmlessly. Heavy drinking, however, tends to waterlog tissues, dilute fluids and impair cellular function. Too much water may also lower the capacity of the blood to absorb and carry oxygen. So don't get carried away!

When I was younger and sillier I attempted to drink 10 litres of water in one day! Why you may ask, as did many others? My answer was, 'Because I can'. Well, I couldn't! After about 9 litres and water running out of my nostrils I thought I should stop! For the next few days I felt terrible. It is not something that I recommend you try!

What Type of Water Should I Drink?

What **type of water** should we drink? There are generally three categories of thirst quenchers we reach for. I will list them in order from lesser to greater preference:

- Water substitutes – juices, soft drinks, coffee, alcohol etc

- Tap water

- Pure, filtered or bottled water.

Many people have got into the habit of thinking that anything with water in it is as good for them as water. While it is true that beer, coffee and soft drink all have a high percentage of water, it is also true that the other ingredients in them may cause a variety of negative responses. In particular one that we are specifically trying to avoid by drinking, which is dehydration.

Tap water is a very common source of water. But even tap water is not necessarily the best option. Tap water is a chemical cocktail. It contains pollutants from the environment and chemicals that are deliberately added in an effort to purify the water and kill bacteria. Unfortunately these chemicals are more harmful than the bacteria they are supposed to kill. Even the fluoride added to the water to strengthen our teeth is not in the form that the body can use for that intended purpose.

The best option is purified water. Bottled water is a good emergency resource, but not something I would base my water drinking around. Why? For a start there are limited regulations on the quality of bottled water and you can really never be sure of what you are getting. The other thing about bottled water that people rarely consider is the ongoing cost. We only spend a couple of dollars here and there, but we never really stop and think about the overall cost. Maybe you should stop and think about it. Let's say a family of four spends $30 a week on bottled water. Over ten years they will have spent $15 000. Was that your jaw I heard dropping!?

Here is a much better idea – for a small upfront investment a quality water purification system will not only ensure the qualilty of the water you are drinking, but over 10 years you will save over $10 000. I'll drink to that!

Free Radicals

Before getting into the details of vitamins and minerals I would like to briefly discuss a substance that is the major cause of disease. This substance is called the free radical. The free radical is accidentally formed during a chemical reaction in the body where oxygen is reduced to create energy. Free radicals are mainly oxygen molecules with at least one unpaired electron. These are very unstable molecules and will try to gain an electron from any substance or molecule in the vicinity. Whichever part of the body recives the most free radical damage will wear out first and potentially develop a chronic degenerative disease.

Chronic degenerative disease includes coronary heart disease, cancer, stroke, diabetes, arthritis, eye disease, Alzheimer's, Parkinson's disease, multiple sclerosis and rheumatoid arthritis to name a few. In fact Dr Ray Strand, MD, suggests that free radical damage is responsible for over 70 chronic degenerative diseases of the modern era. Free radicals are generated through a variety of activities and situations, including:

- Air pollution

- Water pollution

- Soil pollution

- Smoking

- Ultraviolet sunlight

- Excessive exercise

- Excessive stress

- Burnt foods

- Medications and radiation.

As you can see, almost without exception, free radicals are impossible to avoid.

Let's talk briefly about cigarettes. What you put into your body is your choice, but please consider the consequences. Smoking not only creates serious health risks for the person intentionally inhaling the smoke but can affect other people (non-smokers) who are breathing it in without realising it.

I am not here to get on my soapbox, but while I am up here: if you are considering quitting, please give it up for everyone's sake.

The only way we can fight free radicals is by eating foods or taking quality natural supplements that contain anti-oxidants. Anti-oxidants neutralise the effect of free radicals, protect cells and therefore reduce the risk of specific diseases. Many vitamins, minerals and phytochemicals are powerful anti-oxidants. These will be revealed as we progress.

Vitamins

All living things, plant or animal, need vitamins for health, growth and reproduction. Vitamins are used as tools in processes that regulate chemical activities in the body and that use carbohydrates, fats and proteins to form tissue and to produce energy. They are good guys.

There are 13 different vitamins that have been identified: A, eight B-complex, C, D, E and K. These vitamins are classified into two groups: fat-soluble and water-soluble vitamins. The fat-soluble vitamins (A, D, E and K) do not dissolve in water and are absorbed and digested in a similar manner to fat. The water-soluble vitamins dissolve in water and include the B group vitamins (see later).

With the exception of vitamin D, which the body can make from sunlight, and vitamin K, which can be supplied by organisms in the large intestine, the body is unable to make vitamins. They therefore must be supplied through food or supplements.

Many vitamins work together to regulate several processes. A lack of any vitamins can upset the body's internal balance and inhibit one or more metabolic reactions.

Vitamin A

Vitamin A (for 'Amazing') is a champion for the growth and repair of tissues and bone development. It is great for vision; in fact, Superman eats a lot of vitamin A! It is essential for the proper functioning of most body organs and the immune system. Vitamin A is a powerful anti-oxidant. Food sources include cod liver oil, cooked eggs, sweet potato, raw carrot, cantaloupe, spinach, apricot, zucchini and squash.

Vitamin B

Vitamin B (for 'Beauties') complex is made up of eight super vitamins grouped together because of their similar properties and because they have a lot in common and get on really well! They are all essential in facilitating the metabolic processes of the body and so are crucial in many respects, as you are about to see.

Vitamin B1

Vitamin B1, or thiamine, is the inspirational leader of the pack. It leads by example by helping to convert carbohydrates into energy and helping in the metabolism of protein and fats. It is essential for the normal functioning of the nervous system, muscles and heart. Food sources include lentils, peas, long grain rice, wheat germ (can be prone to rancidity and consequently free radical production if not fresh), lean pork, Brazil nuts, pecans, cooked spinach, orange, cooked egg and cantaloupe.

Vitamin B2

Vitamin B2, or riboflavin, is second in charge and a leader in its own right. It is needed for producing energy from foods. It aids in the formation of antibodies and red blood cells and is necessary for the maintenance of good vision, skin, nails and hair. What a star! Food sources include cooked egg, almonds, salmon, chicken, beef, steamed broccoli, steamed asparagus, steamed spinach. Steaming helps to retain more of the nutrients – much can be lost in the water if food is boiled.

Niacin

Niacin (and they don't come any niacer!) is a vital cog in the B team wheel. It is important for the release of energy inside cells. It aids nerve function, energy production and reduces high blood pressure. Food sources include organ meats, lean chicken, turkey and beef, salmon, lentils, beans, peas and tuna.

Vitamin B6

Vitamin B6 is a prime mover in the team and is involved in the metabolism of proteins, carbohydrates and fats. It helps maintain a strong immune and nervous system, aids in the removal of excess fluid in premenstrual women and is great for the skin. Food sources include banana, avocado, salmon, lean turkey and chicken, liver, beef, pork, egg, cooked spinach and vegetable juice cocktails.

Vitamin B12

Vitamin B12 is an all round great vitamin that functions in all cells, but especially in those of the gastrointestinal tract, the nervous system and the bone marrow. It helps to form and maintain red blood cells and is necessary for carbohydrate, fat and protein metabolism. Food sources include clams, mussels, crab, salmon, beef, roast chicken and turkey, and poached eggs.

Folic Acid

Folic acid, otherwise known as 'Fabulous Folic' is necessary for DNA and RNA production, which is essential for the growth and reproduction of all body cells including the formation of the red blood cells. Food sources include liver, soy beans, broccoli, cooked spinach, cooked asparagus, cooked lentils, cooked garbanzo and lima beans and fortified cereal.

Biotin

'Big Bad Biotin' helps to break down carbohydrates and build other super compounds from protein and fats, such as healthy hair. Food sources include liver, soy beans, fresh wheat bran, cooked eggs, chicken, pork, salmon, avocado, raspberries, cooked artichoke and raw cauliflower.

Pantothenic Acid

Pantothenic acid performs a plethora of prime purposes! It participates in the release of energy from foods. It helps in development of cells, the central nervous system and the immune system. Food sources include liver, kidney, tinned tuna, chicken, cooked egg, yoghurt, steamed broccoli, lentils, split peas, sweet potato and raw mushrooms.

Vitamin C

Vitamin C (for 'Colossus') is essential in the formation and repair of bones, skin, teeth, tendons and supportive tissue. It is a main player in the prevention and fighting of infections and colds. It aids in the absorption of iron. Vitamin C is a powerful anti-oxidant. Food sources include orange and orange juice, grapefruit and grapefruit juice, strawberries, tomato, sweet red pepper and broccoli.

Vitamin D

Vitamin D (for 'Darn Good') promotes the absorption of calcium, which is important for the normal formation of bone, teeth and cartilage. The skin forms vitamin D when exposed to sunlight, but may need more from food sources including cod liver oil, salmon, canned shrimp and sardines, and fortified cereal.

Vitamin E

Vitamin E (for 'Exceptional') helps to form and protect body tissues. It supplies oxygen to the blood, which is then carried to the heart and other organs. Vitamin E is a powerful anti-oxidant. Food sources include olive oil, soy oil, canola oil, safflower oil, sunflower oil, almonds, spinach, carrot and avocado.

Vitamin K

Vitamin K (for 'Kan't do without it'!) assists in clotting of the blood. Food sources include olive oil, soybean oil, canola oil, cooked broccoli, raw spinach, raw lettuce, raw watercress and raw parsley.

Minerals

No, I'm not talking about eating rocks! Most fresh and natural foods contain minerals and, like vitamins, they are vital for the normal growth and function of your body. Many people these days consume a large proportion of highly processed foods and they are missing out on the majority of important minerals that can only be supplied through fresh foods. This mineral deficiency, as with vitamin deficiency, may lead to very serious health consequences.

There are two kinds of minerals: **macro** and **trace**. Macro means 'large' and so your body needs larger amounts of macro minerals. Trace means 'small' and so your body needs only small amounts of trace minerals.

Macro Minerals

Calcium
Helps to form strong bones and teeth, aids muscle function, blood clotting, nerve function and reduces blood pressure. Food sources include milk products, dark green leafy vegetables, broccoli, shrimp, salmon, clams, legumes and tofu.

Chloride
Helps with fluid balance, acid-base balance, digestion and is part of the acid in the stomach. Food sources include salt and most foods, especially prawns and olives.

Magnesium
Helps in the development of bones and teeth, to transmit nerve impulses, in muscle contraction and the activation of enzymes, and is needed for energy. Food sources include wholegrains, nuts, legumes and dark green leafy vegetables.

Phosphorus

Helps to form strong bones and teeth, acts as a buffer in maintaining the acid–base balance, helps to transport fat and process carbohydrates. Food sources include brains, liver, sardines, meat, eggs, poultry, milk products, legumes and nuts.

Potassium

Helps with fluid balance, transmission of nerve impulses and the making of protein. Food sources include dried fruits, kiwifruit, stone fruits, avocados, legumes, meat, vegetables, bananas, milk and fruit.

Sodium

Helps to maintain and regulate fluid balance and acid–base balance, and helps the transmission of nerve impulses. Food sources include salt.

Trace Minerals

Chromium

Is essential for converting glucose (or sugar) to energy. Food sources include meat and wholegrain cereal.

Copper

Is needed for production of haemoglobin, helps make red blood cells, strengthens blood vessels and helps with other enzyme functions. Food sources include organ meats, shellfish, legumes and nuts.

Fluoride

Helps with the formation of bones and teeth and the prevention of tooth decay. Food sources include toothpastes and seafood.

Iodine

Essential for manufacturing thyroxine, the thyroid hormone. Food sources include seafood and iodised salt.

Iron

Helps to produce haemoglobin, which carries oxygen from the lungs to the body. Food sources include red meat, organ meat, egg yolk, legumes, enriched cereals and bread, green leafy vegetables and dried fruits.

Manganese

Works with enzymes to help with many cell processes. Food sources include wholegrains, nuts, fruits and vegetables.

Molybdenum

Works with enzymes to help with many cell processes. Food sources include organ meat, cereals and legumes.

Selenium

Has anti-oxidant properties, works with vitamin E and helps with normal muscle function. Helps to remove toxins from the body. Food sources include seafood, meat and wholegrains.

Zinc

Activates enzymes for important functions, helps in the production of insulin and the making of sperm, is an anti-oxidant and helps in the prevention of cold and flu. Food sources include meat, poultry, fish, eggs, wholegrains, legumes and nuts.

Phytochemicals

Phyto means plant in Greek, so the term phytochemicals refers to naturally occurring chemicals found in plants. Whether or not phytochemicals are essential has not been determined, however, numerous studies show that a high intake of fruit and vegetables can lower the chance of developing diseases such as heart disease, cancer and cataracts. It certainly won't hurt to eat these foods and will quite likely improve overall health so it's got to be worth it.

The following table outlines the types of phytochemicals, their food sources and possible health benefits.

Phytochemicals	Food Sources	Possible Health Benefits
Carotenoids	Orange pigmented and green leafy vegetables, carrots, tomatoes and spinach	Anti-oxidant, antimutagen, anticarcinogen, enhance immune function
Flavonoids, isoflavonoids and saponins	Green and yellow leafy vegetables, parsley, celery, soy beans, and soy products	Anti-oxidant, anticarcinogen, has similar properties to oestrogen
Polyphenolics	Cranberry, raspberries, blackberries, rosemary, oregano and thyme	Anti-oxidant, antibacterial, reduce urinary tract infection
Catechins	Green and black tea	Antimutagen, anticarcinogen
Isothiocyanates and indoles	Cauliflower, brussel sprouts, broccoli and cabbage	Antimutagen
Allyl sulphides	Garlic, onions and leeks	Anticarcinogen, antibacterial, cholesterol lowering

Terpenoids	Citrus and caraway seeds	Anticarcinogen against breast tumours
Phytosterols	Pumpkin seeds, sunflower seeds and soy beans	Reduce symptoms of prostate enlargement
Curcumin	Tumeric	Anti-inflammatory
Salicylates	Grapes, dates, cherries, pineapple, oranges, apricots, gherkins, mushrooms, capsicums and zucchini	Protects against large blood vessel disease
L-dopa	Broad beans	Used in the treatment of Parkinson's disease
Non-digestible carbohydrates	Artichoke, chicory root, murrnong, maize, garlic, oats, fruit and vegetables	Stimulate growth of potentially useful bacteria in gut, cholesterol lowering

Just in case you don't know what some of the above terms mean, here are some definitions:

- Anti-oxidant – a substance that counters the effect of cancer-causing free radicals.

- Anticarcinogen – a substance that counters the action of a carcinogen (cancer agent).

- Antimutagen – a substance that counters the effect of a mutagen (an agent contributing to cancer by damaging DNA).

Summary

Okay, well there it is: water, vitamins, minerals and phyto-chemicals in a nutshell. I hope you can see the importance of these quiet achievers. When planning your menu ensure that you include the fresh foods that contain them. They are crucial if your goal is optimal health and disease prevention.

To be more specific I encourage you to include the following foods in your day-to-day eating:

- Wholegrain foods

- Nuts and legumes

- Leafy green vegetables

- Avocados

- Seafood

- Most fruits and vegetables

- Anti-oxidants – tea (especially green), red wine (in moderation), extra virgin olive oil (in moderation), vegetables and fruit.

Supplementation

I hope that you have taken this chapter on board and are now committed to eat more fresh fruit and vegetables. If for some reason your eating is lacking in any of the major nutrients, vitamins or minerals then I would recommend some quality supplements. Look for a brand that is all natural, possibly organic and that is totally plant-based so that the phyto-chemicals are still present.

Even if you do eat fresh fruit, vegetables, fish and meat, supplements are still worth considering. Have you ever thought about what happens to food before you buy it?

Most conventional farms grow crops in nutrient deficient soils, thus producing nutrient-deficient plants. Pollutants in the air, pollutants in the water, pollutants in the soil, pesticides, and chemicals added to preserve the life and look of fruits and vegetables will all detract from the food you purchase. Animals are fed nutrient-deficient plants and are treated with hormones and antibiotics, and food is treated with additives and pollutants before we eat them. Processed foods contain synthetic fats and carbohydrates as well as other additives including preservatives, colours and flavour enhancers. The major deficiencies and problems associated with this are the loss of many vital vitamins, minerals and phytochemicals by the time the food gets to your mouth, and increased free radicals released in the atmosphere and in our bodies.

To make sure you are getting the required nutrients that are crucial to optimal health, I recommend you source quality, natural supplements that include:

- A daily multi-vitamin and multi-mineral tablet

- Anti-oxidants – vitamins A, C and E (these will be included in a quality multi-vitamin supplement)

- Omega 3

- Others you may need for specific deficiencies, for example iron, calcium, magnesium, selenium.

Here are the last two things I am going to say on supplementing:

1 Look very seriously into it and get more information.

2 Don't settle for cheap synthetic supplements that are readily available.

Remember you are looking for a product that will improve the quality of your life, help you to live longer and prevent chronic degenerative disease, so don't compromise quality for cost.

Taking synthetic supplements is just like eating synthetic and processed foods – they are not going to supply you with the nutrients in the form that your body can identify or use. Think about this. The money you spend now on quality organic and natural plant based supplements will save you much more on disease treatment in later life. Not to mention the increased enjoyment, satisfaction and achievement you'll experience.

Supporting References

Savige, Dr G. et al., *Agefit* (2001), Pan Macmillan Australia.

Diamond, H. & M., *Living Health* (1988), Transworld Publishers, USA.

Walker, Dr R., *The Cell Factor* (2002), Pan Macmillan Australia.

Strand, Dr R., *What Your Doctor Doesn't Know About Nutritional Medicine May be Killing You* (2002), Thomas Nelson, Inc. Nashville, Tennessee, USA.

8
Shopping for Success

Well, we know what sort of food we need to be eating and when. The next step is to know where to get it, which types and brands are best, who to believe and how to know which product contains the best ingredients.

This really can be a difficult process. As mentioned earlier, manufacturers want to sell their products and so will appeal to the consumers' needs. Most shoppers want food that tastes good and is good for them, others just want food that tastes good.

Shopping and food selecting is fraught with dangers. The supermarket is like a big spider web where the unsuspecting consumer will wander in and fall prey to the clever yet deceptive marketing of many products with so-called health benefits.

When you walk into the supermarket and see 99 percent fat-free ice cream, 97 percent fat-free rice crackers, 98 percent fat-free breakfast bars, low cholesterol margarines, low calorie jams and diet yoghurts, what do you think? 'GREAT, I can have great-tasting food that won't make me fat'. Or so you believe.

Let's do a little exercise before I get into this too much further, just to get your mind working.

Which Would You Choose?

What follows is a nutritional information chart comparison which represents three food products. Your job is to read and compare the chart for each product and decide which one you would buy. I will then give you some more information.

Breakfast Cereal

Nutritional Information	Product A (per 100g)	Product B (per 100g)
Energy (kJ)	1543	1252
Fat (g)	6.4	2.5
Carbohydrates – total (g)	71	73
– sugars (g)	15.2	18.5

Snack Fruit Tubs

Nutritional Information	Product A (per 100g)	Product B (per 100g)
Energy (kJ)	120	324
Fat (g)	0.08	0.1
Carbohydrates – total (g)	7.3	18.5
– sugars (g)	6	14.5

Soy Milk

Nutritional Information	Product A (per 100g)	Product B (per 100g)
Energy (kJ)	185	175
Fat (g)	0.8	3.2
Carbohydrates – total (g)	12	10
– sugars (g)	4	2

Okay, so based on that information which product for each food would you choose, A or B?

Here is some more information for you. What follows is the ingredient list for each of the above products. Do they confirm your decision or confuse you? Keep in mind that ingredients are listed in order of quantity: greatest to least.

Breakfast Cereal

Ingredients	Product A	Product B
	Rolled oats, sultanas, Triticale flakes, wheat flakes, barley flakes, peaches, apricots, apples, sunflower kernels, sesame seeds, cinnamon	Sultanas, rice flakes, malt, wheat bran, emulsifier (471), glucose powder, wheat, bran flakes, liquid malt extract, salt, honey, preservative (220)

Fruit Snack Tubs

Ingredients	Product A	Product B
	Diced peaches, water, artificial sweeteners (952, 954), anti-oxidant (300), food acid (334)	Peach, fruit juice, vitamin C

Soy Milk

Ingredients	Product A	Product B
	Soy protein, maltodextrin, sugar, food acid (332), mineral salts (341, 452) emulsifier (471), vitamins, water	Organic whole soy beans, canola oil, sea canola oil, salt, salt, filtered water

What do you think now? Has reading the ingredients, and knowing what you now know, caused you to change your mind on any of the original choices?

Would it be fair to say that most people make a decision about a product based first on the amount of fat, second the amount of calories and third the amount of carbohydrates?

If we are going to read a label, the first place we generally look is the nutritional information chart and just take the numbers on face value without looking deeper into the source of the figures.

This is something I will go into in more detail in this chapter, and I will give my preferred selection for the above products. Until then we have got some work to do. Are you ready? Good! I will separate shopping for food into three categories: (i) natural fresh foods (ii) packaged natural foods and (iii) packaged processed foods.

Natural Fresh Foods

I recommend that as much as possible you choose fresh and natural foods in preference to pre-packaged and processed options. There are some exceptions to this, which I will cover in due course.

The first decision you need to make is whether you want to go with standard fresh food or organic produce.

Organic food is a far better health option. Organic produce is grown without chemicals, pesticides, preservatives or other additives. Organic meats are raised without hormones, antibiotics and other chemicals. The benefits are food that tastes great, offering long-term health and reduced risk of many diseases which are increasingly commonplace.

On the negative side, organic food will cost considerably more due to limited supply and specialised production. It will be harder to find, again due to limited supply. Organic food will not last as long because it is not treated with chemicals or preservatives. Consequently its appearance may be less than perfect. If however, you can overcome these minor inconveniences, organic food is your best option. In Chapter 9 I will go into more detail of the benefits of organic produce.

Your fresh-food shopping list should include:

High GI fruit: Watermelon, cantaloupe and pineapple (for times when you need to get your blood sugar levels up or to combine with other low GI fruits).
Low GI fruit: Apples, pears and mandarins, etc (see Appendix) for snacks and adding to meals to reduce overall GI.
Fresh vegetables and salads: Buy a variety of vegetables. Use for stir-fries, salads, sandwiches, snacks, soups, etc. It is okay to buy some higher GI produce as long as you have enough low GI ingredients to counter their effect.

Sweet potato: Instead of potato, parsnip and pumpkin.

Fresh nuts, seeds, olives and avocado: Yes, higher in fat but a healthy fat. These foods are good for you in moderation. The best nuts are almonds, walnuts and macadamias – unsalted and unroasted of course! Use avocado in salads or as a spread instead of butter or margarine. Olives can be used in salads and others dishes.

Fresh and lean meat and chicken: Choose very lean cuts with the fat removed. Free-range chicken is also an option.

Lots of fish: Especially deep-sea fish and those higher in Omega 3 fats, e.g. salmon, sardines, tuna, trevally, perch, blue eye, blue grenadier, snapper.

Eggs: Use only one or two yolks at a time, with as many whites as you like. Look for the omega 3-enriched eggs.

Packaged Natural Foods

Some pre-packaged fruits, vegetables and proteins can be quite a healthy and convenient option. Make sure that there is no added sugar, salt or other chemicals and additives. These products are:

- Some frozen vegetables

- Some tinned fruits and vegetables

- Some tinned or packaged tuna and salmon.

Packaged Processed Foods

Generally speaking, if it comes in a box, a bag, a tube or a can it has been processed and contains some chemicals or artificial additives. This is how the product can stay on the shelf for so long. In addition, much of the food's nutritional goodness has been lost in the production and packaging process.

The most important thing you can learn about making the best selection is how to read labels and decipher the information given on the packages. You will often be sidetracked and influenced by the obvious message that the manufacturer is trying to get across.

Be very wary when the following words or statements confront you:

- 98 percent fat-free (or some other low-fat advertising)

- Lite

- Diet product or Low Joule

- Cholesterol free

- Used and recommended by a sporting celebrity or association.

When I say be wary, I mean that these recommendations or so-called benefits don't necessarily mean that it is either a healthy product or one which will help you achieve your goals.

The nutritional chart given on all packaged produce is useful, but can also be misleading. Misleading because we generally only use it to see how much fat and how many calories are in a product. Is this true for you? In many instances the product that is lower in fat or calories is not the best option. It is the make up of the fat, carbohydrate or calories that will give you a much better indication as to the nutritional value of the food.

Let's have another look at the two breakfast cereals I introduced earlier in this chapter:

Nutritional Information	Product A (per 100g)	Product B (per 100g)
Energy (kJ)	1543	1252
Fat (g)	6.4	2.5
Carbohydrates – total (g)	71	73
– sugars (g)	15.2	18.5

I would bet a lot of money that 99 percent of people, who didn't know better, would choose product B. Would this have been your initial choice?

The reason is obvious; product B has less fat and less kilojoules (calories) per 100g. We have been brainwashed by highly reputable people to keep away from fat and that the more calories we eat the fatter we will get.

What I want to put to you is this: just because a product has more calories, more carbohydrates and/or more fat doesn't necessarily mean that is the least preferable choice. You need to look further into it. You need to go beyond the surface.

This is where the ingredients list comes into the picture. If you can analyse this list in an informed way you can make a considered decision that will lead to the enhancement of health (and taste) and not its detriment.

What you are looking for are ingredients that are natural, low GI, include healthy fats and are free from additives (the numbers).

Let's have another look at the ingredient lists:

Ingredients	Product A	Product B
	Rolled oats, sultanas, Triticale flakes, wheat flakes, barley flakes, peaches, apricots, apples, sunflower kernels, sesame seeds, cinnamon	Sultanas, rice flakes, malt, wheat bran, emulsifier (471), glucose powder, wheat, bran flakes, liquid malt extract, salt, honey, preservative (220)

What do you think now? I hope you have been swayed back to product A, if this wasn't already your first choice. Remember that the ingredients are listed in order from greatest to least quantity.

Product A

The first ingredient is rolled oats, a natural low GI grain.
Sultanas are a moderate GI dried fruit.
Triticale is a very low GI grain.
The cereal is sweetened with real fruits (sultanas, peaches, apples and apricots). There is no added sugar.
The higher amount of fat is made up from healthy fats, i.e. oats, sunflower kernels and sesame seeds.
A good high fibre, low GI and naturally healthy choice.

Product B

Ingredient number two, rice flakes, is an extremely highly processed and high GI food.
Ingredient number three is malt, not just a processed sugar, but also one with a GI of 105, the highest GI!
Ingredient number five is glucose powder, the second from top of the GI tree.

Out of the 12 ingredients, four are moderate to high GI sugars: malt, glucose powder, liquid malt extract and honey.

The cereal contains artificial additives, emulsifiers and preservatives. I will talk more about these a little later.

The small amount of fat this cereal contains is quite likely to contain trans-fatty acids.

A high GI, highly processed cereal and one that I would be avoiding if I were you.

What do you think? Are you starting to understand the vital importance of gaining knowledge of the ingredients listed on packaged products? Product B, by the way, had a name suggesting it was a 'lite' choice for breakfast and advertised as low in fat – a sure seller!

Ingredients – What to Look For and What to Avoid

The list of ingredients will always give you a more accurate indication of the food's value and effect. You should be looking for ingredients that are natural, generally less refined, moderate to low GI, low in trans-fatty acids and saturated fat and that include some healthy fats.

The ingredients are always listed in order of quantity, with the greatest quantity listed first. Foods that are listed way down in the ingredients list will only occur in quite small amounts. This means that you may get away with certain foods if healthy ingredients outnumber them.

Sugar and fat can be included in many forms. Be aware of the different types of fats and avoid foods with large amounts of processed sugars, carbohydrates and fats (see below).

Fats

Yes, we are generally looking for foods that are low in fat. But this statement can be dangerous if taken too literally (as illustrated in the Product A/B example). We need to be aware of the type of fats involved and their effect, positive or negative on health and longevity. In many cases the product with the higher percentage of fat is the better option.

Trans-fatty acids are the ones we specifically need to avoid. Obviously I am not suggesting that you give up all the foods you enjoy, if they contain trans-fatty acids. I am however suggesting a significant reduction in the consumption of these foods. I will be suggesting some healthy and delicious alternatives.

Natural saturated fats should be enjoyed in moderation; this may mean a reduction for some people.

Foods with monounsaturated and polyunsaturated fats are, as we now know, very healthy fats and need to be included in a well balanced eating plan.

When reading the nutritional information labels on packaged food with relation to fat content, be ready to decipher information not given to you directly. Let me explain this statement by giving you two examples.

The following nutritional information label comes from a popular crispbread.

Nutritional Information Per 100g

Energy (kJ)	1640
Fat (g)	
– saturated	1.2
– trans	0.0
– polyunsaturated	3.0
– monounsaturated	5.4
– TOTAL	9.6
Ingredients:	Grains (89%) [wheat, corn, poppy seeds, linola seeds, canola seeds, rye, barley, sunflower kernels, soya bean], sunflower oil, salt, sugar

This label is great and all fat is accounted for. It leaves nothing to the imagination as every type of fat and quantity is clearly shown. As you can clearly see the majority of the fat is made up from monounsaturated and polyunsaturated fats, only a small amount of saturated fats and no trans-fatty acids. Although the fat content is 9.6 percent, I would still consider this a healthy choice, as the ingredient list would confirm. All information is given so you can make this decision with confidence.

The next label you are about to see does not give all the fat information.

This nutritional information label comes from a brand of semi-processed chicken slices.

Nutritional Information Per 100g

Energy (kJ)	512
Fat (g)	
– saturated	1.2g
– TOTAL	3.5g
Ingredients:	Chicken breast, water, salt, mineral salts (451, 450), hydrolysed vegetable protein, preservative (223), vegetable oil, sugar

The difference here is that we know that total fat per 100g is 3.5g and we know that 1.2g of that is saturated, but what about the other 2.3g? This is about 66 percent of the fat content conveniently not accounted for. Why? Let's deduce the reason together. Looking at the ingredient list, would you expect any of the fat in a processed meat product to be monounsaturated or polyunsaturated? A minimal amount if any – so if you thought no, you would be pretty much right. So what does that leave? Did you think trans-fatty acids? Right again. It is only 2.3 grams per 100, but remember a 2 percent increase in consumption of trans-fatty acids may contribute to a 93 percent increase risk of heart disease not to mention the effect on cell membranes.

Be suspicious of any information not supplied on the food label, learn to read and analyse the ingredient list and remember that manufacturers of food are not going to leave off any information about how their product can increase your health!

Types of Fat to Be Enjoyed in Moderation
Oils – flaxseed, olive and fish
Nuts – almonds, macadamias, walnuts
Seeds, avocado and olives
Fish – salmon, tuna, mackerel, sardines, trevally, trout
Lean chicken and red meat
Omega 3-enriched eggs

Types of Fat to Avoid in Large Amounts
Shortening
Lard
Margarine
Butter
Vegetable oil
Copha
Coconut oil
Palm oil
Cocoa butter
Vegetable fat
Hydrogenated vegetable fat
Peanut oil
Canola oil
All animal fat and chicken skin
Processed fats in foods such as muffins, doughnuts etc. and most take-away foods, even so called low-fat products.

Carbohydrates and Sugars

The main problem with the carbohydrate figure on the nutritional chart is that it only refers to the amount of carbohydrates and doesn't differentiate between the types of carbohydrates nor their effect on your blood sugar levels.

You are much better off choosing a product with a higher amount of carbohydrate if that figure is made up of natural, low GI and less refined ingredients.

The same applies for the amount of sugars. There are many types of sugars and you need to understand the impact of these sugars and how the combination of ingredients contributes to the overall Glycemic Index.

Types of Sugars to Avoid in Large Amounts
Glucose

Sucrose

Lactose

Malt/maltose/malt extract

Dextrose

Sugar-raw, brown, cane

Molasses (unless eating for its iron content)

Honey and golden syrup

Rice syrup

Caramel

Types of Refined Carbohydrates to Avoid in Large Amounts
White flour

Wholemeal flour

Rice flour

Corn flour

Choose foods sweetened with fruit, fruit juice concentrate, fruit purée and fructose.

Choose food with less refined carbohydrates such as rye flour, triticale, rolled oats, bran, soy flakes, beans, nuts.

Other Ingredients to Be Aware Of

Artificial Additives

These include preservatives, colourings, sweeteners, thickeners, flavour enhancers, food acids, emulsifiers, anti-oxidants and mineral salts. Watch for a lot of numbers in the ingredient list – these refer to artificial additives.

So that you understand the detrimental effect of these additives let's have a look at some numbers specifically mentioned in our sample products:

Additive	Name	Possible Danger
Preservative 220	Sulphur Dioxide	Can be fatal to asthmatics, destroys vitamin B1 in food, causes gastric irritation and may affect kidney/liver function
Preservative 223	Sodium Metabisulphite	Reduces vitamin B1, gastric irritation, nettle rash and swelling
Antioxidant 300	Ascorbic Acid	Large doses can result in tooth decay, diarrhoea and kidney stones
Food Acid 334	Tartaric Acid	Causes gastric irritation
Mineral Salts 450, 451, 452	Sodium, potassium and phosphates	Disruption to metabolism of calcium/phosphates, linked to kidney stones
Emulsifier 470	Magnesium Stearate	Can irritate bowel lining and skin

| Sweetener 951 | Aspartame | May cause headaches and hyperactivity |
| Sweetener 952 | Cyclamic Acid | Potential carcinogen – banned in UK and USA |

Some additives have potentially severe effects and we need to appreciate that even seemingly healthy ones e.g. anti-oxidant (300) which is L-Ascorbic Acid (vitamin C) is potentially unsafe. It is added not for our health but as a preservative and appearance enhancer. There are several books around that list additives and their effects, and are available at most popular book stores.

Genetically Engineered (GE) Food

GE is a new technology that manipulates the genes and DNA blueprint of living things. Genetic engineers use viruses, bacteria and a device called a gene gun to randomly move genes from one organism into another.

In the genetic engineering of food, these techniques are used to make plants grow differently. For example, a gene from an arctic flounder fish was added to the DNA of tomatoes in order to make the tomatoes resist the cold. Clearly, this would never happen quickly through natural evolution.

By inventing new life-forms in this way chemical companies hope to find new and profitable uses for living things – to alter nature to better suit the needs of industry.

There are serious concerns about the safety of consuming GE foods. There is the possibility of developing antibiotic-resistant bacteria in our bodies, the potential exposure to unexpected proteins, toxins and allergens, and a greater level of pesticides in our food. A major concern is that to this point GE foods have not been tested on humans. Some have not even been tested on animals, therefore their effect is unpredictable and largely unknown.

There is also the possible effect on the environment. Some critics claim that GE crops may contaminate surrounding GE free crops (by cross pollination).

GE ingredients are commonly found in such items as bread, pastries, snack goods, baked goods, vegetable oils, margarine, flours, starches, sauces, fried foods, soy foods, lecithin, sweets, soft drinks and sausage skins. Chickens, cows, sheep and cows fed with GE grains means that fresh meat, milk and eggs may also be affected.

Foods labelled 'Product of Australia' are mostly GE free. However foods labelled 'Made in Australia' may contain imported GE ingredients. Many products do not declare GE ingredients. You should actively choose foods labelled 'GE-free', 'Not Genetically Modified', 'Certified Organic' or 'Certified Biodynamic'.

The good news is that for all the manufactured products high in processed ingredients, artificial additives or genetically modified there are usually plenty of alternatives. By using the information here you can make educated choices of foods and ingredients for meals. A simple rule is to go for foods as close to their natural form as possible.

Do you recall the three products I introduced at the beginning of this chapter? Based on the information you have just received, which **breakfast cereal** would you now choose? If you said **product A**, you are on track. If you said product B, you had better read it all again!

The best **fruit tub** option was **product B**. While product A has fewer calories it is full of artificial ingredients. Product B is much more natural.

My **soy milk** preference is **product B**. Even though it has more fat its ingredients are far more natural and healthy.

Supporting References

Greenpeace, *The Food Guide, How to Shop GE-FREE*, 2nd edition (2003).

Treffers, S., *Food Additives* (1999), Hartrade, Australia.

9

Organic Versus Non-Organic

What's the big deal about organic food? It looks bad, it doesn't last as long and it is expensive! Why should I waste my hard-earned dollars on it?

Good question. Let me try to answer it.

While I briefly touched on organic produce in Chapter 8, I decided it was important enough to warrant its own chapter. So please read this chapter with care and an open mind.

I spoke in Chapter 7 about the importance of vitamins, minerals, phytochemicals and water in addition to quality carbohydrates, fats and proteins in ensuring optimal health. It is a deficiency in these nutrients coupled with a higher consumption of synthetic foods and chemical additives that has, in a significant way, contributed to the alarming rate of many of the modern-day degenerative diseases such as cancer, heart disease, diabetes, osteoporosis and asthma.

Back in the dark ages, primitive people were free of all of these modern day afflictions. Sure, those people were eaten by dinosaurs and had big rocks fall on their heads but their bodies had abundant nutrients! Why? Because they had not discovered chemicals, preservatives, pesticides, herbicides, fungicides, antibiotics and all the other pollutants that now fill our air, our water, our soil, our crops, our food and consequently our bodies.

Primitive people ate plants and berries that had grown in pure, nutrient-plentiful soils. The meat they ate was from animals that had also eaten the healthy plants, or other healthy animals. The water they drank was untouched by artificial additives or pollution, and the air they breathed was fresh and clean.

In a Perfect World

Paul Chek in his book/CD pack *You Are What You Eat* describes the 'Wheel of Life'. Simply put it explains the cycle of life and nutrients from plant to animal to humankind to soil and back to plant.

In a perfect world, plants grow in soil that is nutrient-rich and devoid of any pollutants. The pests are controlled through natural means such as ladybugs and birds, and fertilisation occurs naturally through the decomposition of natural matter. The soil is turned and aerated by earthworms. The plants and soil receive water that is free from pollutants, further enhancing the health of the plant.

Animals feed from the healthy, nutrient-rich plants and drink the pure and plentiful water. They grow naturally and with optimal health; their only major concern is predators, of which humans are one.

The humans eat the natural, nutrient-rich plants and the flesh from the healthy animals. Their bodies grow strong, function well and are able to fight off any infection or other disorder with ease before it can become a long-term problem. Full of energy, the humans are more motivated, more productive and they lead longer, more fulfilled and happier lives. Eventually they invent the TV with remote control and couldn't be happier!

As the plant and animal life die they decompose to further enrich the soil. They create an environment for the earthworms to survive, thrive, turn and aerate the soil. The worms help to create compost, which is ideal food for the microorganisms in the soil which provide the nutrient-rich food for the plants.

And the cycle repeats.

How Did Things Ever Get So Bad?

The population expanded, technology exploded, the demand for food and consumables grew, the need to produce more food at a faster rate created a need for processing, preserving and modifying foods. Chemicals were added to plants to make them grow faster, bigger and stronger. Chemicals were added to the soil and plants to kill and deter pests, or to fertilize the soil.

Unfortunately, what was not considered was that all these chemicals were and still are killing all the vital micro-organisms and essential nutrients in the soil, and leaving nothing but a barren lifeless soil full of harmful chemicals to be passed on to any plant grown in it, and consequently to any animal eating it.

Now consider the modern day 'Wheel of Life'. Plants grow in soil that is nutrient deficient thus producing plants that are nutrient deficient. Chemicals, insecticides, fungicides and fertilizers added to plants and soil further create very undesirable produce. The crops are nourished with water that contains a variety of environmental pollutants, chemicals and bacteria.

The farmed animals are fed these grains and plants and consequently become nutrient deficient and affected from taking in a variety of chemicals. This affects the growth and health of the animals. They get sick and so are treated with antibiotics and other synthetic medications, which not only kill infection but also affect the quality of the muscle (which we will eat). Many animals are kept under inhumane conditions and fed synthetic supplements to enhance growth to cater to the growing demands of the marketplace.

We humans now consume these plants and animals that are in such a bad state and as a result we lack energy, have trouble staying in shape, we are more prone to disease, we spend more time and money at the doctors and the quality of our life is seriously affected. The worst news is that we are less motivated, less productive, achieve less and therefore take a lot longer before we can afford the big screen TV with the remote control!

Conventional Farming (Non-Organic)

Today a large percentage of all of our food is farmed in such a way that the negative 'Wheel of Life' is created. So the fresh produce that looks so good on the supermarket or green-grocer shelves is hiding its history of neglect and poor up-bringing.

But how can fruits and vegetables look so good? The answer is simple – they are treated with preservatives and other chemicals to look enticing to the consumer.

Have you ever noticed how fresh foods are gradually losing their taste? Have you ever wondered how strawberries, toma-toes and other fruits and vegetables can grow so large? Have you ever noticed how you can get fruits and vegetables all year round, even though they are not always in season? The answer to all of these questions lies in the farming process, the state of the soil and the use of artificial means and modi-fications to create more products bigger and faster.

Organic Farming

Organic farmers wish to provide you with plant foods as nature intended. That is, grown in a soil full of all the essential nutrients, using only chemical-free and natural pest controls, and not artificially treated to make them look better, grow bigger or last longer.

Organic meat comes from animals that are allowed to develop and roam as naturally as possible. They are fed only organic food to ensure they grow naturally and disease free.

Certified organic farms must go through a lengthy process to ensure that the soil is totally free from all chemicals, contains all the essential nutrients and is rich in the micro-organisms necessary for the healthy growth and development of all plants. It may take between three and five years to achieve this certification. From that point strict and regular tests are done on the farm and the quality of the soil to ensure standards are being maintained. A similar process is enforced on all organic animal farming.

Taste the Difference

Do yourself a favour. Before you make the decision to change to organic food, do a taste test. Take a certified organic and a non-organic sample of some different fruits, vegetables and meats and taste the difference – you won't go back.

Is It Worth It?

This is a decision only you can make. Before you make it you should consider a few things. Firstly, organic shops and produce are becoming more and more commonplace and consequently the quality is improving and the cost is decreasing. Secondly, when you look at your bank balance and are listing your priorities for spending, is health and quality of life for yourself and your family on the top of that list.

Is it worth a few extra dollars a week to feel better, be healthier and prevent a degenerative disease that could cripple you or a member of your family? Is it worth a few extra dollars to help ensure that the time you and your family spend on this planet is positive, productive and enjoyable? What could be worse than wasting years of your life in doctors' practices, in hospital beds, on operating tables or in bed at home? Would you rather spend your money on holidays, cars, TVs, time with family, your house – or medical expenses, pharmaceuticals and other necessities of bad health?

Thinks about it this way – the time and money you spend now on your health will save you thousands of dollars and give you much more time to enjoy life in the long run.

I have one more piece of advice before you head out on your organic shopping spree. Make sure that the produce you are buying is **certified** organic. It will tell you on the packaging. If it isn't, don't bother – food advertised as organic that isn't certified may well be grown without having been treated with pesticides, herbicides, fungicides or other chemicals. The soil, however, may be affected from previous years of damage and maltreatment and will still pass this on to the plants and consequently to you.

Now get out there and get organic. You will be glad you did.

Supporting Reference

Chek, Paul, *You Are What You Eat* (2002), A Chek Institute Production, USA.

10
The Exercise Factor

How many times have you said to yourself, 'I really need to start an exercise program' but never followed through with it? How many times have you started and stopped an exercise program in a relatively short space of time? Why?

Is part or all of the reason for this behaviour pattern due to a belief that getting any benefit from an exercise program requires a large amount of time, effort and money? More than you are able or willing to spend?

If I were to say to you that you could get fantastic results with your health, strength, fitness and body shape and size without (i) hating the process (ii) spending a fortune (iii) devoting seemingly endless hours and (iv) buying expensive and complicated equipment, would you believe me? I hope so, because I speak the truth!

It is true that if you want to get great results long term out of your exercise regime then, as with anything in life, a consistent effort is required. However, for most people two to three hours per week is all the time that is needed. In terms of equipment and cost, a pair of appropriate shoes, some comfortable clothes and an open mind are the keys to your new body and the start of your new life.

Exercise need not be an experience you hate. You don't need sophisticated equipment or hours of free time. All that is necessary is the knowledge of what to do, and how hard and how often exercise should be done.

I know what you are saying to yourself right now: 'If I am changing the way I eat, why do I have to exercise as well?'. Good question!

The answer is simple: you don't have to do anything you don't want to do!

There has to be a big **however** after that statement, and there is ... HOWEVER, once you understand and are aware of the many benefits from regular exercise you may think differently.

> If you don't feel like you can cope with changing your eating and introducing an exercise program all at the same time, that is okay. Initially focus on the food, then when you have established some good habits and are feeling more energised and more motivated, gradually you can implement the exercise plan.

Whenever you look at someone who exercises regularly you are observing the most obvious physical benefits of this exercise. For a lot of people the main motivation for taking on an exercise regime are the aesthetic benefits:

- Reduction of body fat

- Increase in lean muscle tissue (i.e. the toned look)

- Increase in cardiovascular fitness (e.g. the ability to run to the bus without puffing, or to work if you miss the bus!)

- Increase in strength

- Increase in muscle size (if that's a goal)

- Increase in energy levels

- Improvement in skin and hair condition

- Postural improvement

- Flexibility improvement.

Many physical benefits of regular and varied exercise are not obvious to the observer; they are, however, crucial to living a healthy, functional and happy life:

- Decrease in blood pressure, bad cholesterol and blood fats (triglycerides)

- Increase in core and joint stability and therefore a reduction of pain or injury caused by a lack of this stability

- Reduced risk of heart disease, diabetes and other serious medical conditions

- Improved sleep patterns

- Increased ability to recover from injury and illness

- Increased range of joint mobility

- Improvement in brain chemistry (being happy!)

- Increased muscle strength

- Increased metabolism, which in turn will increase the rate at which your body burns fat

- Increased muscle endurance

- Improved range of joint movement

- Improved bone density

- Improved ability to complete daily tasks

- Improved sporting performance (indoor or outdoor!).

These many physical benefits promote a variety of positive associated effects:

- Increase in self esteem and self image (i.e. confidence)

- Reduction in stress

- Increased social participation (i.e. meeting new people)

- More consistent moods

- More productive (in all areas of life)

- More fulfilling relationships (due to more energy)

- Greater life achievements

- Greater enjoyment of life.

Even if you experienced only a small number of the benefits listed above, wouldn't your world be a better place?

The intention of this chapter is to show you that great results can be achieved by including some regular enjoyable exercise in your life, and that getting great results from exercise need not require a huge time or effort commitment – just consistency. I will aim to give you some important guidelines and things to consider, including how your newly acquired eating knowledge and regime will fit in with your exercise.

How Much, How Long, How Hard?

When you start an exercise program, I'm sure your intentions aren't to go for a short period of time and then stop. Yet for most people this is exactly the case. In fact of all people who join a gym, only about 10 percent of them will still be exercising regularly 12 months later. Of the people who discontinue exercising, the vast majority will give up within the first three months!

Think about the reasons why you may have stopped an exercise program in the past. Do they include any of the following?

- Boredom

- No enjoyment

- Lack of variety

- Lack of knowledge of what to do

- Perceived lack of results

- Results not happening fast enough

- Time

- Weather

- Soreness or injury

- Fatigue

- Too busy

- Money

- Lack of correct equipment

- Inability to maintain the regime

- Personal issues (e.g. relationship break up)

- No one to exercise with

- An event in your life (e.g. pregnancy, new job, moved house)

- Perception that you are too old

- You don't get on with your trainer

- The program doesn't work.

I'm sure there are many more reasons that you have experienced or heard of. The question is, and you have to be truly honest with yourself here: 'Are these legitimate and justifiable reasons for me to stop exercising?'

If the answer to that question is yes then this chapter should help to guide you in dealing with the particular issue or issues.

If the answer is no, then the greatest realisation that I can hope to pass on is that you, and no one but you, are responsible for the outcome. The sooner you take responsibility for your actions the sooner you will start on the track that leads to long-term success.

Furthermore, there is no tablet you can take to make you fit! There is no electronic zapper machine that you can attach to your problem areas to tone your body! There is no abdominal apparatus that you can use for only five minutes per day that will make your body look as good as the models advertising it.

In fact the only benefit of purchasing any of these products is that if you do so within the first 15 minutes of the ad being shown you get the steak knives as well!

Okay, now I've got that off my chest, let's look at the things you must consider before you begin. The aim is to develop new habits that will last a lifetime and create balance, happiness and fantastic results.

Remember this: any exercise program will work if it is followed consistently and to the appropriate level.

Questions to Ask Yourself

The very first question you must ask yourself before starting any regime is: 'Can I maintain this long term?' If the answer is no then my advice is don't even try or chances are it will become another failed attempt. To ensure a lifetime commitment to exercise make sure you can answer yes to the following questions:

1 ***Do I really want to start an exercise regime?***
This must be a decision made for the right reasons – because you really want to change, not because someone said you should.

2 ***Am I prepared to commit to this long term?***
You need to understand that you are about to go through a lifestyle change for a lifetime, not just until summer! You need to understand that there are no quick fixes (that last) and be willing to take as much time as is necessary to change your thinking and consequently gain the body and life you desire.

3 ***Do I enjoy the exercise I am doing?***
If you don't enjoy it, no matter how hard you try, it won't last. Find some exercise that you enjoy and can enjoy the benefits of.

4 ***Is there enough variety?***
Variety will increase your enjoyment and motivation and your body will benefit in many ways from a range of exercise styles and techniques.

5 ***Is the time commitment maintainable?***
You will be told many things about how much time you need to commit to exercise. Before you believe everything you hear, keep this in mind – anything more than

you are doing right now will have a positive effect. Make sure you start with a modest and realistic approach and then increase.

6 *Have I made my exercise regime a priority in my life?*
To be successful with your training it has to be done consistently. This means the times you allocate for exercise must have a high priority and other commitments must be arranged around them.

7 *Am I doing appropriate exercise for my goals?*
If you are trying to lose body fat then, as good as it is, doing yoga three times a week is not the most effective way to achieve this goal. Make sure you understand what is the most effective and enjoyable exercise for your needs.

8 *Am I doing the appropriate exercise for my level?*
Don't expect to improve if you are exercising at a level that is below your ability. On the other hand don't try to maintain a level that is beyond your capabilities.

9 *Am I progressively increasing the intensity and/or workload of my exercise?*
Insanity is doing the same thing over and over and expecting a different result. If your goal is to continually improve then, as you adapt to your exercise, you need to gradually and progressively increase the load until you get the level that you are happy to maintain.

10 *Am I keeping a record of my exercise?*
Documenting all the exercise that you are doing will help you set goals for the next sessions and ensure that progressive improvement occurs.

11 ***Am I giving myself adequate recovery?***

Recovery and rest is just as important for your body as exercise. This is where your body and mind recuperates, regenerates and rebuilds – muscle strength and energy systems adapt and improve during these recovery periods.

12 ***Am I eating appropriately?***

Need I say more? Regardless of how often and/or how well you think you are exercising, you will struggle to achieve long term results if your eating is not complementing your exercise regime.

Find a Friend

You may not know how to recognise or apply some of the above considerations. If this is the case then I would strongly suggest that you involve someone else in this process. Find a knowledgeable friend or a fitness professional to at least get you started on the right path. To head off in the wrong direction is sure to end in tears!

A good personal trainer or health/fitness mentor will help you to:

- Identify what you want to achieve and set effective goals.

- Create an enjoyable exercise plan that suits your lifestyle.

- Teach you how to exercise at the appropriate intensity for your goals, age and level.

- Encourage a gradual increase in effort and intensity.

- Explain the importance of balance, variety and recovery for achieving your long-term goals.

- Ensure that your technique is sound and that good posture is always maintained.

- Identify areas that need extra attention, e.g. flexibility, joint and core stability.

- Keep you accountable for achieving your goals.

- Push you when you need to be pushed and know when you need to rest.

- Create a balance in other areas of your life.

- Keep you on track with your eating.

- Encourage, support and mentor you.

- Be a friend.

- Answer any questions you may have about exercise, food, injuries or any other related issues.

The right person is someone with whom you have a rapport and can have some fun as well as be serious about your goals. Use the above list as a checklist in your selection process.

Types of Exercise

Exercise is a very general term and refers to many types of physical exertion. A balanced and effective exercise regime must include some percentage of each of the following:

Cardiovascular Exercise

This type of exercise involves strengthening the heart and lungs. It increases your overall fitness level, and is the type of exercise primarily responsible for fat burning.

Strength Exercise

The aim is to increase muscle strength, size and endurance. It also increases the body's metabolism and consequently its ability to burn fat.

Stability Exercise

This is a type of strength training. It involves strengthening of the muscles responsible for core (lower back) and joint stability. Pilates and yoga include this type of exercise.

Flexibility

Flexibility involves increasing muscle elasticity and joint mobility. It's important for good posture, injury prevention and rehabilitation, increased performance and general wellbeing. Yoga includes a high degree of flexibility work.

The Fun Stuff

As well as enjoying all the above, it is important to include things you love to do. For example, tennis, golf, squash, dancing, footy, cricket, rock climbing, mountain bike riding, hiking and many other sports and leisuretime activities. All have great health and happiness benefits.

Rest and Recovery

This is a vital part of any exercise regime. It allows muscles to recover, regenerate and rebuild, and it allows for psychological recovery and ongoing enthusiasm. Rest and recovery ensures that each exercise session can be completed to the best of your ability ensuring maximum effect.

How you incorporate each piece of the exercise puzzle into your regime really depends on your needs, goals and time restraints. It is quite possible that several of the above components may be combined into one session to make it a much more time efficient process.

Get your mentor, personal trainer or fitness professional to help you:

(i) Develop the plan incorporating the above areas.

(ii) Implement an exercise regime that suits your goals, your current fitness level and fits in with your present lifestyle.

(iii)Monitor, re-assess and modify your program on a regular basis.

(iv)Create an enjoyable routine that will continue to provide great results and that you feel is maintainable for the rest of your life.

Eating and Exercise

At this point I want to make one point very clear. You may be at a stage in your life where many areas need to change for you to enjoy your existence for as long as possible. Please don't feel that you have to make all these changes at the same time. I am specifically referring to changing your eating patterns and introducing an exercise regime: two major life-altering decisions.

If you honestly feel you can do both and maintain them, then I say go for it. If you have some doubts about introducing too many changes at once and maintaining them, then I say don't even try.

Your first priority should always be your eating regime. Get that right and it will be much easier to introduce exercise. If you have optimal energy through quality nutrition you will be motivated to exercise regularly and to a level that will promote positive change.

On the other hand, if you attempt to introduce exercise into your life without first addressing your nutrition you will find it difficult for many reasons. A lack of energy will result in a higher rate of missed exercise sessions, and will reduce the level to which you can exercise and hence the results which you could achieve.

If you are of the opinion that the more exercise the better, without increasing your nutritional intake, you are likely to be messing with your metabolism and therefore reducing your body's ability to burn fat. Introducing exercise without addressing nutrition is more likely to leave you with less energy than before, and make you more irritable, less able to deal with stress and generally not a nice person to be around. Exercising without properly replenishing your body's energy systems will severely affect the results you can achieve and the way you look and feel. There is a higher likelihood of craving and consumption of the wrong type of food at the wrong time of the day.

All of the above reasons create a situation that you are specifically trying to avoid by exercising in the first place.

Develop an enjoyable eating regime, increase your energy levels consistently and then introduce the exercise.

Eating To Maximise Exercise Effect

To ensure you get the maximum effect from your exercise, the way you include food into this process is vital. Historically the common belief has been that to lose weight it is important to exercise more and eat less. I hope that, from what you have learnt from this book, you can appreciate how this is the worst possible strategy if long-term results are the goal.

Here is the outline of a sample day of healthy and high energy eating without any exercise. After I have discussed the three main aspects of eating and exercise I will show how you can fit exercise into the plan.

7am	1 slice watermelon
7:20am	1 bowl natural muesli with skinny milk, strawberries and natural yoghurt
9:15am	1 apple
11am	2 Vitaweat biscuits with avocado, tuna and tomato
1:15pm	Salad – chicken, lettuce, tomato, avocado, cucumber and sweet potato or chicken, avocado and salad sandwich on rye bread
3:30pm	10–15 nuts (almonds, walnuts and macadamias) and 1 apple
5:30pm	1 tub natural yoghurt
7:30pm	1 salmon steak with stir-fried Asian vegetables

Three aspects of eating and exercise are crucial: pre-exercise, during exercise and post-exercise. To neglect any of these would compromise your efforts to exercise optimally and minimise the benefits.

Pre-Exercise

Regardless of the time of day that you prefer to exercise, eating beforehand is crucial to ensure maximum energy.

If you are training at any time other than first thing in the morning then follow these guidelines: the closer you can comfortably eat to your exercise routine the better your energy levels will be. Fruit is a good pre-exercise food to eat close to exercise as it is easy to digest and will help to maintain your blood sugar levels at their optimum level.

If you train first thing in the morning, it is even more important to eat something. At this time of day your blood sugar levels are very low and need to be raised. Not eating at this time, as many professionals suggest, will put you well 'behind the eight ball' in terms of your energy levels and your ability to exercise to your potential. Starting the day with low blood sugar will have negative effects on hunger, cravings and the body's tendency to hang on to fat as the day progresses.

The early morning eating plan still applies. That is, eat a high GI food followed by a low GI food. Because you are training, these need to be easily digestible foods. Let's say you train at 6:30am. Get up at 6am and eat a small amount of watermelon. Ten to 15 minutes later eat a handful of grapes or drink orange juice. The goal is to raise blood sugar levels and then stabilise and maintain them into the exercise session.

During Exercise

Depending on the type and duration of exercise, I recommend including an intake of energy throughout the session. The aim of this food is to enable you to keep performing at your maximum throughout the session.

If it is a high intensity exercise or lasts longer than 60 minutes you should be prepared to eat or drink throughout. For example, long bike rides, long runs, sporting games with breaks.

The food needs to be of moderate GI and easy to eat and digest. Try bananas, bars, drinks (e.g. sports drinks, juice, watered down cordial). High GI foods and drinks can be used in this situation but they need to be consumed at regular intervals to ensure blood sugar levels don't drop too far.

Post-Exercise

The 20 minutes after exercise is the time when your body is most receptive to nutrition in terms of energy replacement, muscle regeneration and recovery, and ensuring metabolism increases.

There are generally three types of sessions you will partake in:

1 Cardio only

2 Strength only

3 Cardio and strength combination.

The post-exercise eating will vary slightly for each.

Directly after a cardio session or a strength and cardio session (i.e. within five minutes) you need to consume a high GI food or drink. This is to replenish energy stores and raise the blood sugar level. The best option in this situation is again watermelon or a sports drink.

Within the next 15 minutes a substantial low to moderate GI food or meal is required. If strength work was a part of the program then this meal should include protein. The carbohydrate in this meal will continue to replenish energy stores and maintain blood sugar levels. The protein is required for muscle recovery and regeneration. Try natural muesli with strawberries and yoghurt, toast or a sandwich with egg, ham, chicken or tuna, basmati rice with chicken, or a protein and fruit smoothie.

After a strength-only workout a moderate GI meal including protein is required within 20 minutes. The carbohydrate will replenish energy stores and the protein will regenerate and feed the muscles. See examples above.

This pre- and post-exercise eating is to be included in your eating plan at the time of the day that the exercise suits you most. To give you some idea of how you may do this, have a look at the same eating plan I outlined earlier with the exercise sessions and extra eating requirements included. It's important to note that I am not suggesting that you do these three sessions in one day – this is simply illustrating how you may include any one of those into various times of your day.

The sections highlighted show what you may eat around an exercise session, whether it's an early morning run, a lunchtime weight session or an after-work, pre-dinner weights and cardio session.

6am	1 slice watermelon
6:15am	**a handful of grapes or a glass of orange juice**
6:20–7am	**RUN**
7:05am	**1 slice watermelon or sports drink**
7:20am	1 bowl natural muesli with skinny milk, strawberries and natural yoghurt
9:15am	1 apple

11am	2 Vitaweat biscuits with avocado, tuna and tomato
12–12:45pm	**Weights workout**
1pm	**fruit and protein smoothie**
1:15pm	Salad – chicken, lettuce, tomato, avocado, cucumber and sweet potato or chicken, avocado and salad sandwich on rye bread
3:30pm	Nut mix (almonds, walnuts and macadamias) and 1 apple
5:30pm	1 tub natural yoghurt
6–7pm	**30-minute weights session followed by 30-minute bike ride**
7:05pm	**1 glass of sports drink**
7:15pm	**1 protein shake**
7:30pm	1 salmon steak with stir-fried Asian vegetables

The protein shake may not be required if dinner is eaten within 15–20 minutes of the sports drink.

Summary

Let me again emphasise how important it is to eat to complement your training. Consider the three following scenarios:

1 Exercising regularly without considering eating. The consequences will be:
   - Losing some weight (possibly muscle)
   - Getting fitter, but lacking energy
   - Having difficulty removing body fat
   - Feeling even more tired than normal – affecting all areas of life
   - Craving sweet or high fat foods
   - Difficult to maintain.

2 Eating well, but no exercise. You will achieve:
   - Increased energy
   - More productivity
   - More consistent moods
   - Reduced cravings
   - Losing body fat and feeling better.

3 Combining your already-established eating plan with a regular exercise regime will give you:
   - Increased energy
   - Greater fitness and strength levels
   - Much more productivity
   - Greater metabolism
   - Leaner and more toned
   - More motivated to take chances and be challenged in all areas
   - Greater achievements
   - More positive outlook on life
   - Much more.

Obviously scenario 3 is the long-term goal. Scenario 2 can be used as a stepping stone to ensure that you are able to enjoy the benefits for the rest of your life. And Scenario 1 must be avoided!

11
Eat Chocolate and Drink Alcohol

Okay, this is the stuff you have been waiting for! Forget about GI, forget about exercise. When does the chocolate and alcohol come into the picture?!

I have just received an email from one of my clients and had to laugh. It was headed: 'Chocolate is a Vegetable' and then proceeded as follows:

1 Chocolate is derived from cocoa beans. **Beans = vegetables**.

2 Sugar is derived from either sugar cane or sugar beets. Both of them are plants, in the vegetable category.

3 Thus **chocolate is a vegetable** and a healthy food!

Well, I'm convinced!

Isn't it amazing how we can justify the consumption of certain foods when we believe deep down that we shouldn't be eating them? It happens all too often and is usually followed by tremendous guilt and consequently one of two responses:

1 **The 'I've eaten fish and chips and drunk beer, I must pay' response**. This involves getting up the next day and running 10km, riding for one hour, doing 100 push ups,

500 sit ups and then fasting for the next three days. This continues until all memory of that weak moment has passed!

2 **The 'I'm a failure, I can't be disciplined so why even bother' response**. This involves giving up trying to give up 'unhealthy bad foods' and binge eating just to compound the fact that you really are a failure.

These two responses have one thing in common. The decision-making process by which they are both formulated is an emotional one. I will discuss this in greater depth as we progress. But first I want to talk about the word **health**.

Complete Health

When referring to all foods we generally give them a label: good or bad, healthy or unhealthy. Celery is a 'good' food, chocolate is a 'bad' food – so we have been told. Carrot juice is 'healthy', beer is 'unhealthy' – or so we believe.

When we use the word healthy, particularly in relation to food, we are generally referring to its effect on our physical state.

My strong belief is that to be healthy does not just mean to be absent of physical disease or affliction. When using the word healthy we must consider not just physical health, but also psychological, emotional and spiritual wellbeing. To not respect all aspects of overall health is a serious oversight and one that can only lead to an individual lacking the ability to live and enjoy life to the fullest.

Case Study: Sue

With this very special case study I'd like to demonstrate that the physical is very much determined by the mental, emotional and spiritual, and that all four contribute to overall health.

My mother, Sue, the greatest inspiration in my life, was diagnosed with breast cancer in 1988. Some time after an operation to remove this cancer it reappeared in her liver and is still there today. Since the time of her initial diagnosis Sue has been through countless forms of treatments and changes from radiotherapy to many varieties of chemotherapy to natural treatments, to eating changes, lifestyle changes and changes of attitude towards her life and her mortality.

The bottom line is that she has an amazing attitude, an incredible will to live and is as tough and persistent as they come. Every time she has a bad blood test or scan she deals with it and moves on to the next plan, the next treatment and the next path to life and happiness.

Many would say that because she has cancer in her body she is not healthy. I will dispute that until all breath has gone from my body. She is now one of the healthiest people I know. Since the time of her diagnosis she has made some life-altering changes. She has learnt to relax, meditate and handle stress. She has learnt the negative effect that guilt has had on her life and has been able to resolve relationship issues that have influenced a major part of her existence. She has developed a deeper and stronger love for her husband, Bill, and her gorgeous children! She has learnt to deal with a life-threatening condition and make the most of her life. She travels, socialises, exercises regularly and eats well and is, with the exception of having the cancer in her body, as happy as she has ever been.

Room for Indulgence

I love a beer as many people do! In fact there are times when I drink too many and get a bit silly. I know that physically, drinking beer is one of the worst things that I can do for my body. I also know that after a hard week of working and training there is nothing better for my state of mind than to go out with friends, drink some alcohol, unwind and relax. I consider it to be one of the most enjoyable aspects of my life and a healthy thing to do. I wouldn't give it up.

Obviously if I drank excessive amounts of alcohol on a regular basis it would undoubtedly and negatively affect my health in most of the four areas. But I don't. I enjoy it in moderation and I make sure that I am consistent with my eating so that my body can easily deal with the alcohol that I drink.

I hope the point that I am making is clear: there IS room in everybody's life for indulgence and foods that are commonly labelled as 'bad' or 'unhealthy', as long as a consistent and balanced way of eating is followed.

It is unhealthy to try to deprive yourself of these foods as it will create a world of stress and disharmony for yourself and those close to you. The end result of this type of existing (not living!) is very likely to be:

- A feeling of loss of control

- A tendency toward binge eating

- The possibly of eating disorders

- A negative emotional state, and serious self-image and self esteem damage.

Step One: Change Your Way of Thinking

The first step to arresting this situation is to change the way we label and perceive food. We must stop identifying and labelling food as 'good or bad', 'healthy or unhealthy', 'junk' and so on. Why? Because this label is then transferred to us as soon as we decide to consume that particular food – 'If I eat that 'bad' food then I am a 'bad' person'.

These labels are referring only to the food's effect on our physical state and don't take into account the positive effect that the moderate amount of this food has on our overall health and wellbeing.

If we do something we think we shouldn't be doing it is generally followed by one of the most destructive emotions there is: GUILT.

Close your eyes and think of all the foods you really enjoy, but either avoid or feel really guilty about eating because of their label. Let's call it the 'pleasure' list. Does it include any or all of the following?

- Chocolate

- Alcohol

- Pizza

- Ice cream

- Fish and chips

- Cakes, biscuits and pastries

- Fast-food

- Lollies and soft drinks

- Cheese

- Chips, nuts

- Butter, oils and margarine

- Eating out.

You will be told by many people, ranging from doctors to 'health' professionals to friends and family, **not** to eat these foods because they are bad for you. Let's be totally honest here, if you were told to never eat these foods again, would you take the advice? If I wrote in this book that you had to give up eating and/or drinking all of the above foods what would you think? You'd think I was an idiot and you would probably use this book as a fire starter! In fact I'd think I was an idiot!

If you enjoy the above 'pleasure' foods you should be able to eat them and still get the results you would like. So step two in this process is to understand the concept of moderation and balance.

Step Two: Moderation and Balance

Develop an eating plan for yourself, similar to the one described in Chapter 4. Make sure you include foods that you enjoy, foods that will achieve the blood sugar objective and foods that you can consume when you need them most.

Make sure this is a plan that you can maintain, and take the time to establish it as a normal routine in your life. This is your base eating plan and should be followed consistently for the majority of the time. I recommend that, to start with, you try to implement the plan from Monday to Friday as it is easier to structure a regular routine on weekdays. Then allow yourself some indulgence on the weekend.

Within your basic and consistent eating plan it is imperative that you allow yourself to eat and drink the foods from the 'pleasure' list and enjoy them.

I would like to re-emphasise at this point that it is a mistake to try and make massive changes in a short period of time. If you consider yourself a chocoholic and eat it every day, then don't attempt to cut that back to once a week in the next week. Remember anything you do better than the week before will have a positive effect on all areas of your health. So take it step by step. Rather than going from eating chocolate seven times a week to once a week, go to five times a week, then four, then three and so on. Take manageable steps, and only take the next one when you are emotionally and psychologically ready.

Step Three: The Decision-Making Process

The next crucial step involves your decision-making process. When you decide to indulge, you should totally understand the reasons for your decision, as they will give you a direct indication as to your state of mind and hence the quality of your overall nutritional consumption.

Let's say you decide to eat some chocolate. This decision, as with any, requires a weighing up of the pros and cons, for example the taste factor versus the effect on your body. Depending on your state of mind that decision will be either emotionally or logically based.

As hard as it may be, separating the emotion from your decision-making process is vital. Let's have a look at the two processes that may lead us to that decision to eat chocolate:

Emotional: This is generally followed by a life-threatening craving: 'If I don't have some chocolate now I will die!' or 'I can't cope with this situation, I'd better eat some chocolate!'

Logical: This is a carefully considered decision. 'I have followed my eating plan this week and trained well, I feel like and deserve some chocolate and am going to enjoy it.'

The difference is clear. In the first scenario the decision was due to a craving or an emotional response. Think about the reason why you may be suffering from cravings. In many instances it is because you have allowed your blood sugar levels to drop. They are low, your energy levels are low and hence your ability to make the most appropriate nutritional choice is severely reduced.

In the second instance the decision to eat chocolate is not based on a perceived necessity, but as an option and a reward for consistent behaviour. This is a 'healthy' decision made by someone with an understanding that this moderate amount of chocolate will improve their state of mind without negatively affecting their physical state. You need to understand that eating chocolate doesn't mean that you are a failure or lacking willpower or self-discipline but rather that you enjoy a variety of foods and understand the importance of balance and allowing yourself some indulgence. You understand that you can enjoy some indulgence and still achieve great results.

For those of you who believe that you are a 'chocoholic' and that it is an incurable medical condition or genetic malfunction I have good news – this is not true. In most cases, dealing with the reasons that blood sugar levels are low in the first place can control these cravings. That is, making sure that for the majority of the time you are following the guidelines that have been outlined in this book.

You will be amazed and delighted to be able to fly through the afternoon with energy and without those chocolate (or other) cravings that continually seem to thwart your attempts to have a better body forever.

The Final Step: Achieving the Balance

The final step to achieving a balanced life is to know the best times to eat from the 'pleasure' list. This is different for everyone and you need to be comfortable with the lifestyle you have developed for yourself. Indulging too often will have a negative physical effect, and indulging too little will create issues with the other three aspects of overall health.

Here are a few things to consider.

Make a decision as to what you will be comfortable with. Having boundaries is a good way to keep you on track. For example, I might set myself the following weekly goals:

• Alcohol on three days (2 to 4 glasses each time)

• Two chocolate bars

• One night at a restaurant – no limit to eating

• Dessert one night.

By setting myself these limits I have things to look forward to, but in a controlled amount. The weeks may vary a bit – some weeks I may indulge less and others a bit more – but I have a gauge.

As I am getting fitter, leaner and feeling better I am less inclined to want to consume these foods and will naturally develop a healthy balance.

As I mentioned earlier, you can't go from excess to moderation in a short period of time. Set yourself some realistic stages along the way to your ideal lifestyle. Get some help with this if you need to.

Case Study: Bob

In relation to the above point, I have a client whom I see on a monthly basis. He is 50+ years old, overweight and diabetic with heart troubles. We have been talking for about 18 months. In that time we have successfully developed an eating regime that he can maintain. The problem is his alcohol consumption, which was something like 60 to 70 standard drinks per week. His doctor has told him to give up drinking. We have set a monthly goal to gradually reduce total alcohol consumption, in terms of the number of standard drinks. The last time we spoke he was down to 30 to 35 drinks per week, still too much but better than 60 to 70! Each month his consumption is reducing. It may take another year or more, but we will continue until we have found a level he can maintain and which will create a positive health benefit.

There are certain times of the day when it is better to indulge than others. In fact, depending on the consumption time, some foods that would normally not be the best choice can be quite beneficial. Certain high GI foods should generally be avoided, but in terms of energy replacement they can be beneficial first thing in the morning or straight after a strenuous cardiovascular exercise session. For example jellybeans and other lollies, rice crackers, soft drinks. During an active day would be a better time to indulge than in the evening when you are in 'relax mode'. Save the treats for times when you are more likely to burn off the energy that you have consumed.

If you have been consistent with your newly developed eating regime, then it is perfectly acceptable every now and then to say, 'I am going to eat what I want and enjoy it'. Don't worry about the time of day or the effect on your body, embrace your indulgence in the knowledge that it has been well deserved.

All foods have a place in your eating regime. Some should be consumed more regularly and others less regularly. If you are consistent with your approach then you have every right to enjoy your indulgences and to create an enjoyable balance in your life. The key word for this chapter when it comes to indulgences is **moderation**. Follow a moderate approach, remove the emotional aspect and you will learn to love eating, an area of life that many people are afraid of.

12

Dieting – the Dos and Don'ts

This is simple: DO not diet and DON'T diet. See you in the next chapter!

Okay, maybe I need to go into this in a bit more detail. For decades and maybe even centuries (I'm not quite that old) people have been trying to lose weight. In the modern era (the last 20 to 30 years) it has become an obsession for many people.

Why? We all know that being overweight for most people is a physically unhealthy state to be in. But for some people this is not a strong enough motivator to address the situation. One of the things that has the greatest influence on how people view themselves is the media's portrayal of what is the norm.

Every time you open a magazine, every time you turn on the TV, every time you drive past a billboard you are confronted with models, actors and other celebrities whose bodies we look at and accept as the way everyone should look.

Many fashion stores stock only the smaller sizes, compounding even further the negative way you may feel about your body and yourself. There are many gorgeous and thin and handsome and muscle-bound singers, musicians, actors, television presenters and other celebrities out there who really aren't that talented. It really makes me wonder how many extremely talented people are unable to get work or get the break they need because of their physical appearance. This is a sad reflection on our society.

The consequence is that we often attempt to achieve for our body that which is unrealistic and unreasonable. We fail to realise that our body shape is largely pre-determined and though we can reduce our size we can't significantly change the shape. Consequently, years and years of unsuccessful and damaging attempts are made trying to force a square peg into a round hole.

This has lead to myriad marketing and diet product opportunities for people who offer fast results for those desperate to lose weight.

Have you ever been on a diet that has lasted more than 4 to 6 weeks? Do you enjoy your lifestyle when you are on the diet? Do you still enjoy the benefits of any diet you have been on? Would I be wrong in assuming the answer to all three questions is no?

Let's look at a couple of diet examples:

1   The following diet was published in a weekly magazine and promoted as the diet responsible for the awesome body of a well-known actor. See what you think.

Typical Daily Menu

Breakfast   Green coconuts then six glasses of vegetable juice
(yummy!)
Lunch   10 oranges OR
Avocado 'burritos' wrapped in purple cabbage leaves
(I am salivating!)
Dinner   Sprouted buckwheat pizza topped with salty olives and baked in the sun (unless you live in

a cold climate!) OR chunks of fresh raw fish drizzled with olive oil and lemon juice, dressed with sea salt and a touch of radish.

Okay, maybe it was this diet and a lot of plastic surgery that gave this actor her 'svelte and sexy new figure'! Let's be honest – who could stand this diet for more than one day?

2 Another popular diet, The Soup Diet, is so bad for you that it even comes with a description of the symptoms you will experience:
   • Because you're not consuming many carbohydrates, some may find the glucose in their bloodstream becomes too low, causing hypoglycaemia.
   • This can cause a range of symptoms, such as headache, sweatiness, anxiety, irritability and drowsiness.
   • Don't worry, it might sound awful but it's easily fixed.
   • If these symptoms occur repeatedly consult your doctor.

Source: www.todaytonight.com.au

Common Questions About Dieting

Some serious questions need to be answered.

Q: What is a diet?

A: A lot of people will give you a different definition of a diet. In my opinion a diet is a quick fix, fast weight loss, calorie-restricted eating plan. By its very nature it is something that cannot be maintained for long periods. Diets may vary in their appearance but their outcome and long-term effect will always be the same. Please note that some diets are required for medical reasons and certainly have a place.

Q: If diets don't work long-term why do we keep using them?

A: The reasons why we may continue a diet or go back to using a diet that we have previously been unable to maintain may include:

a. The fact that we did lose considerable weight quickly.

b. It works well in the lead up to an event like a wedding or holiday in the sun.

c. The feeling while we are actually losing weight is one of euphoria and is addictive.

d. We blame ourselves because we didn't have the will-power to maintain the diet and so try again.

Q: Whose fault is it when a diet fails?

A: Most people blame themselves because they feel they are weak and have no self-discipline to maintain the diet. However, it is highly unlikely that every single person who ever dieted is weak and lacking in self-discipline! The fact is that the diet had no chance of success. The whole diet concept is self-defeating. When you tell yourself 'I'm going on a diet' it can only lead to 'coming off the diet'. DO NOT blame yourself.

Q: Why is so much weight lost on a diet?

A: This is a question that has been covered in a fair amount of detail in Chapter 2. Due to the severe calorie restrictions of the diet, the body is forced to break down lean muscle for energy. Lean muscle is quite dense and hence carries considerable weight, which is lost during this process. The body will lose a large amount of water when dieting, which also contributes to this weight loss. A much smaller percentage of this weight loss will be attributed to fat loss.

Q: Is weight an accurate indicator of fat loss?

A: When it comes to your scales, my advice would be to use them as a doorstop! They most certainly should not be, in 95 percent of cases, the indicator of your attempts to lose fat. Why not?

When you get on a set of scales you are weighing everything: skin, bones, muscles, blood, organs, food just eaten, waste products, fat, clothes etc.

It is quite possible and highly likely that if you are exercising and eating appropriately your weight will remain constant or even increase while you lose substantial body fat.

On the other hand a decrease in weight can easily be accompanied by an increase in body fat if dieting or calorie restriction is the process.

Weight can fluctuate on a daily basis and have nothing to do with your attempts to lose fat. Hormones, fluid retention, food, bodily functions and many other things can cause your weight to vary up to 2 to 3kg (4 to 7lb) per day.

Q: What is the best measure of fat loss?

A: There are several ways to monitor fat loss:

    a. Regular skin fold measurements, which can be done by a personal trainer, at a gym or other health centre.

b. Tape measurements – these are not the most accurate but are better than scales.

c. The way your clothes fit.

d. The way you look in the mirror, and comments from other people.

One thing I often say to clients who find themselves addicted to scales and desperate for weight to drop is: 'If you look good and feel good then what does it matter what your weight is?'

Q: What about height versus weight charts?

A: My advice is to throw them away. What they fail to take into account is that everyone is different. How can everyone possibly be put in one category? They are dangerous, as I will illustrate. I am about 5'11"; weigh 90kg and my body fat is less than 10 percent. According to the height/ weight chart I should weigh between 65 and 81kg! If I were someone who didn't have a clear understanding of my body and the relationship between fat and weight I would panic and take extreme and unhealthy measures to get my weight down into the 'healthy' range for my height. This is where crash dieting usually comes into the picture.

Q: Why don't diets work long term?

A: Dieting may most accurately be described as starving your body. As we know, the theory is that by severely restricting your calorie intake your body will lose weight. We know that this is true. This serious deprivation has many serious effects on metabolism, mood, ability to function normally, hunger and cravings. No matter how strong-willed a person you are you have to live and your body will only allow so much deprivation before either eating or death prevails. When the eating finally prevails it often comes in the form of bingeing and due to the starvation effect on metabolism, body fat will be stored much more readily and be much harder to get rid of. We therefore find ourselves back at square one or even worse off in a short period of time.

Q: What if I just want to kick-start my weight loss and metabolism with a couple of weeks of dieting and then I will follow a more normal way of eating?

A: This is a question that I get asked regularly. The important point here is that dieting won't kick-start metabolism, it will slow it down. So, in two weeks time, when eating returns to a more normal intake, all the sacrifices made in that two-week period will be totally wasted. In fact the body will be in a worse state than it was at the start of the two weeks, in no time at all.

Q: What are the long-term effects of dieting?

A: The list is long and terrible. Years of starting and stopping myriad diets may contribute to:
- Brain damage
- Liver damage and disease
- Kidney damage and disease
- Decreased contraction of the heart (possible sudden death)
- Short-term memory loss
- Lowering of metabolism
- Loss of lean muscle
- Predisposition to store excess fat
- Irritability
- Reduced ability to function effectively
- Reduced enjoyment of life
- Unhealthy relationship with food
- Development of eating disorders
- Self image issues
- Loss of self esteem and self worth
- Relationship issues with self, family and friends

- Increased stress
- Possibility of life-threatening conditions such as heart disease, diabetes, cancer.

The time to stop dieting and stop looking for quick fixes is now.

Be very wary of any diet or eating plan that:

- Includes the word 'diet'

- Promises quick and easy weight loss

- Claims a breakthrough

- Restricts the foods that you can eat

- Uses a well-known name to imply endorsement

- Promises spot reduction

- Requires an unusual eating style

- Includes meal replacement pills, bars or powders.

Are You Addicted to Dieting?

Answer the following questions to see whether dieting has a hold over you:

- When you try to lose weight do you try to do it quickly?

- Is weight loss on the scales the be-all and end-all for you?

- When you decide to lose weight do you automatically think of dieting?

- Have you attempted dieting 10 or more times in your life?

- If you eat any indulgences while dieting do you feel like you have failed the diet?

- Do you feel guilty when you eat indulgences?

- Are you likely to try just about anything to get your weight down fast?

- Are you scared to eat too frequently because you might put on weight?

If you have answered yes to four or more of the above questions then it is time to start changing the way you think about food. These are issues you need to consider very carefully.

Eating to Lose Fat Versus Starving to Lose Weight

This goes against every dieter's understanding and every diet's philosophy. In order to increase metabolism, maintain blood sugar levels and encourage fat loss most people need to eat much more regularly. The obvious condition here is that we eat the right type of food at the right time of the day.

Short-Term Versus Long-Term Results

Think very carefully about which of the two options is best for you.

Short-term results: Severely restrict your food intake, place your life under much stress, reduce energy levels, avoid going out, be irritable and moody, struggle at work, struggle to exercise, lose muscle, lower metabolism, lose weight for a short time but eventually put it all back on and more with an associated feeling of failure and negative self esteem.

Long-term results: Take some time, learn new habits, be consistent, change you attitude toward food, enjoy the process, be full of energy, eat all the foods you enjoy, keep your metabolism ticking, lose fat, and continue to achieve great things for the rest of your life.

Quality of Life Versus Appearance

Obviously this is strongly related to the issue of short-term versus long-term goals. Is the way you look so important that you will sacrifice and compromise every other area of your life? Is it worth wasting a certain part of your life for a look that you will be unlikely to maintain anyway? Surely life is too short!

Eating the Right Type of Carbohydrates

By eating natural, unprocessed and fresh carbohydrates at the time of the day when your body most needs them you will have the greatest chance of achieving the results you want for the long term. If you understand that all carbohydrates are different and each has a different effect on your blood sugars you will realise that the blanket statement 'carbohydrates make you fat' is an uneducated and short-sighted one. Don't be scared of carbohydrates – use them for good and not evil!

The Emotional Aspect

One thing that you must take some time to work on is removing the emotional aspect from the decisions that you make. Easier said than done. Chapter 13 deals with this highly important and influential aspect of being a happy human.

Summary

DO NOT DIET. I hope I have been clear enough.

Supporting Reference

Cardwell, G., *Diet Addiction* (1994), Wellness Australia.

13
Get Off the Emotional Rollercoaster

We can't ignore the emotional aspect of our lives and the part it plays in the things we do, the things we say, the decisions we make and the food we consume. We are human and the thing that separates us from many other living things is the emotional factor.

Rather than blame our emotions for things we do and say and the position we may now find ourselves in, we should learn more about ourselves. Discover the situations that lead to certain emotions and learn the patterns of behaviour that result. If it is a healthy and happy response then all is fantastic. If the pattern of behaviour is a destructive one then only misery, heartache and unhappiness will result. It is possible, however, to relearn new patterns in response to certain emotions.

I am not a psychologist, but every day I deal with people with emotional and self-esteem issues. One of the most important lessons that I have learnt and can pass on to you is that it is only possible to change physically if you are able to change emotionally and psychologically. That is, change the way you feel about yourself and change the way you respond to the things that happen to you in your life.

It has been said by many great people that it doesn't matter what happens to you, it is how you react to what happens that will determine the final outcome. Not a truer statement has ever been made.

Have a think about a time in your life when something happened to you. Think about your emotional response to that occurrence. Then think about whether your life was better or worse as a consequence of that response. Hindsight is a wonderful thing, but unfortunately at the particular time it's not available. Wouldn't it be great to be able to make the most positive and healthy response to any situation no matter how bad it seems?

Let me give you an example. In the previous chapter I talked about dieting and the magnetic and dangerous effect that the scales have. In a very serious attempt to lose weight by dieting, subject X was horrified on a daily weigh-in to observe that her weight had increased by one kilogram. She felt numbness take over her body. She was confused, angry and upset. Her reaction was a common one. 'This isn't f#&*ing working!' She then proceeded to binge eat. At the conclusion of her binge eating she lay on the couch in tears. She felt guilty for bingeing and a failure for not maintaining the diet. Her self-esteem plummeted. In her mind she felt there was no way she could ever get in the shape she wanted because she had failed so many times, was undisciplined and didn't deserve to anyway.

This is a common response by many people. However, rather than the self destructive path described above, there is a much more positive, healthy and empowering action that subject X could have taken in response to the situation. This I will discuss later in the chapter.

One of the greatest factors in creating long-term change is the ability to love, accept and truly believe in yourself. The many emotional responses to an array of situations will have a profound and ongoing effect on self-image, self-esteem and self-belief. Unfortunately for many people these are largely negative and extremely limiting.

Throughout our lives we are subject to ongoing feedback about the way we look, the way we act and the things we can

achieve. Our parents and family, our school peers, our part-
ners, our work colleagues and many other people influence
the way we perceive and feel about ourselves. We will be told
that we look good or bad, that we can achieve what we want
or not, that we are a valuable person or not. Who are we not
to believe them?

We may have tried on countless occasions to lose weight
and in every case been unable to succeed for the long term.
Rather than learning from the experience we develop the
belief that we are weak and will never truly be as we so des-
perately want to be.

In my position I come across these people every day of my
life. They honestly can't see or believe how good they can be
or what they can achieve. One of the greatest rewards for me
is to help one of my clients realise that they are a valuable
person and that they can achieve what they previously
thought unattainable. To see them grow in stature and confidence and continue to surprise themselves as to what they
are really capable of is why I do what I do.

Strategies

Here are some strategies for making your world a more positive place:

1 **Look for a positive in every situation, no matter how bad it may initially seem.**
A close friend of mine was recently diagnosed with breast cancer and has just had a mastectomy. When I first contacted her after I had heard the news I was expecting depression, confusion and anger. Her response was one of great surprise and pleasure to me. She described the diagnosis as a 'great wake-up call' and is now already planning to make some changes that will make her a healthy and happy person for many years to come. If only everyone in this position reacted in the same way.

2 **Accept yourself as you are.**
This doesn't mean you can't try to improve yourself, but accept where you currently are and love yourself with the knowledge that you are a valuable person. Remember, no one is perfect!

3 **Associate with positive, supportive and encouraging people.**
You are able, for the most part, to choose the people you spend time with. Make sure they accept and love you for yourself and will always help and encourage rather than criticise and blame.

4 **Avoid negative influences.**
In some cases this may be a difficult thing to do because those influences may be family or work colleagues. If this is the case then you may need to confront these people and make them aware that their attitude is a destructive one for you. If they care they will do something about it.

If they don't then they have no place in your happy and productive life.

5   Don't let others criticise you or your body.
What do they know anyway?

6   Learn to forgive others.
Don't hold on to hate, bitterness or resentment. If you can learn to truly forgive others who intentionally or unintentionally harm, you can free yourself of many destructive emotions. Rather than blaming a perpetrator, forgiving them will allow you to move on with your life and not harbour and relive bad situations and all the associated harmful negative emotions.

7   Learn to forgive yourself.
We all make mistakes, we all eat food we feel we shouldn't and we all say the wrong thing every now and then. It is okay, learn from it and move on. If you can forgive yourself you free yourself from one of the most destructive emotions – guilt. Dr Gerald G Jampolsky in his book *Forgiveness – The Greatest Healer of All* defines forgiveness as 'letting go of all hopes for a better past'. Think very carefully about that.

8 Don't be influenced by the media's portrayal of what is the norm.
The fact is that most of the models or celebrities in magazines, on TV or in the public eye are very much out of control when it comes to their bodies and their eating. Eating disorders are commonplace and many celebrities/models are far from happy with themselves. Don't immediately believe the media's perception of the truth until you have looked into it more closely.

9 Recognise negative self-talk.

Catch yourself in the act and find a more positive way to speak to yourself.

10 Focus on the process, not the results.

Getting on the scales every day and hoping that your weight has gone down will only lead to pain and failure. If you have developed an enjoyable plan of eating and exercise and are following it consistently, the results will take care of themselves.

11 Reward yourself for every small step on the way.

For example, if you are trying to eat breakfast each day, then make sure you celebrate and 'pat yourself on the back' each time you do. Each week that you are a little better than the week before is a success even if you may have eaten something you feel you shouldn't have.

12 Your past does not equal your present or future.

Just because you may have tried and failed to lose fat long-term several times in your past, it doesn't mean the next attempt won't succeed. You do, however, need to change your beliefs, attitudes and patterns of behaviour.

13 Involve someone else in the process.

Understand that you will be unable to move on with your life, your body and your happiness if you can't change the way you feel about yourself. Talk to a friend, a mentor or a psychologist and learn to control the emotions that are a roadblock to your happiness.

14 Understand that you, not anyone else, are responsible for your own happiness.

Why Do We Eat?

If we can stop, think about and understand the factors that trigger us to behave in certain ways then we take a large step toward being able to manage behaviour in response to different emotional situations.

I like to separate the triggers for eating into two main categories: the 'Eat or Die' category and the 'Because it is There' category.

Eat or Die

These triggers are based on the body's physiological need for nutrients and energy. We have to eat to live and so the body sends signals for us to recognise when we are in need of nutrition, or in fact when we need to stop eating. Some of the signs to eat include hunger, salivation, lethargy, headaches and cravings. Feelings of fullness and even feeling of illness are signals to stop eating or suffer the consequences.

Because it is There

We are human and as such we interact with many influences. This category includes triggers in our life that we cannot avoid.

Sights, Sounds and Smells

Think about the smell of food, the sight of food in shops and in cookbooks, food advertisements, food in convenience stores and take-away outlets. Think about how products may be advertised or placed on supermarket shelves. Think about the way a packaged product may look, or the song used in the commercial, and how we associate these images/sounds with eating. Think about where convenience stores are located and the introduction of 'drive thru'. Makes it easy and attractive, doesn't it?

Social

Social cues are hard to avoid. Almost every social engagement you will attend will be centred around food and drink. 'Let's go out for dinner', 'Let's catch up for a coffee and cake', rather than 'Let's go for a walk and a chat'. We often fall into the trap of just going along with this rather than suggesting other ways of 'catching up'. Once in a food-oriented social situation, it may be difficult to make your preferred food choices. In many cases it is easier to eat what you would rather not eat than to have to explain why you are not eating what everyone else is. This is an issue that I will touch on in the next chapter.

Emotional

As we well know, our eating habits can be highly influenced by many different emotions. Anger, sadness, happiness, depression, loneliness, frustration, guilt, boredom and envy will cause some people to overeat and others to stop eating. It is a regular pattern that someone eats a certain food as a result of an emotion such as depression. It is just as common for this behaviour to stimulate another emotion, the most dangerous one of all – guilt.

Unfortunately there are no set rules for how a person may react to particular emotional situations. It is important that you are able to identify your own triggers for certain eating patterns. By creating this awareness you are much more able to change your behaviour patterns if they are destructive to your physical being and self-esteem.

Here are some strategies that may help you to cope with, manage or avoid situations that have caused trouble in the past:

- I have already stressed the importance and value of a food diary to monitor energy levels and food intake in terms of its effect on your physical being. If used correctly a food diary can help you to uncover patterns and triggers for eating. Make sure you detail times, places of eating, who with and the emotions before, during and after the meal.

- Visibility of food is a strong motivator for eating. Try to avoid situations where you are exposed to food for long periods of time.

- If certain emotions are a regular cue to eat or not eat, develop a number of alternative coping strategies that don't include food. The more strategies you have, the easier it will be to choose one that is a more appealing option. For example, if your response to being upset is to eat chocolate, then develop some other options such as going for a brisk walk around the block, calling a friend, punching a boxing bag, or screaming really loudly. Remember that, as with anything, it may take some time to develop these new responses into unconscious ones. Make sure you allow yourself this time and strongly deter yourself from your usual destructive pattern while the new patterns are established.

- If you are a reflex eater then try to distract yourself from food until you are able to make a conscious decision to eat. Most urges to eat, unless caused by genuine hunger, do not remain consistently strong; they only last while the conscious thought is in your mind.

- Don't allow yourself to get over-hungry. This is a point that I have already emphasised. It is almost impossible to ignore the cues if you are really hungry and your blood sugars are low.

- When you get that strong urge to eat, rather than focusing on how you feel at that point, try to visualise how you will feel after you have eaten.

- If you do overeat or eat something that you would have preferred not to, don't punish yourself. Remember you are human, no one is perfect and it is okay to indulge every now and then. Punishing yourself will more likely lead to negative self-esteem and an unhealthy cycle of eating.

It is not easy to change your emotional responses and cues for eating, but once you do, you will experience a profound effect on your life. Again I strongly recommend getting some help in this area if you don't feel you can cope on your own.

Scenarios to Avoid

The following is a list of possible scenarios that could cause a destructive emotional reaction, along with my suggestions for a more positive long-term response.

Scales

Showing a weight increase or no change.

Common emotional and physical reaction(s):

- 'I'm getting nowhere' or 'I am going backwards'.

- Give up, binge eat and eat badly again, or further restrict food intake and train more.

Positive long-term response:

- Understand that weight and fat loss are not necessarily related.

- Understand that scales are a bad indicator – clothes or body fat measurements are more appropriate.

- Focus on the process not the results.

Increase in Body Fat

Common emotional reaction(s):

- 'I'm no good, I can't do it, what is the point?'

- Give up or take on an unhealthy and unrealistic eating and exercise regime.

Positive long-term response:

- Use it as a learning experience. Find out the reasons why it happened and make some gradual changes to ensure it doesn't happen again.

Wanting to Lose Weight Quickly

For example, for an upcoming event or for summer.

Common emotional reaction(s):

- Go on a restrictive diet.

- Overtrain.

- Partake in some quick weight loss scam.

- Compromise health and long-term results.

Positive long-term response:

- Slow down.

- Take the time to develop good habits, change thinking and attitudes.

- Sacrifice your ultimate look this year and make the effort to be in the best shape for next year and every year after.

Traumatic Episode

Such as death, relationship split, work stress.

Common emotional reaction(s):

- Not hungry, can't eat so don't eat.

- Feeling of sadness, anger, worthlessness, rejection and/or guilt.

- Bingeing and overeating.

Positive long-term response:

- Find a positive in the situation, no matter how hard it may seem.

- Understand that you will cope better with all stresses if you follow the appropriate eating plan.

- Don't blame yourself.

- Change your response and association to cues that normally produce negative and destructive patterns of behaviour.

History of Carrying Too Much Fat and Yoyo Dieting

Common emotional reaction(s):

- Focussing on long-term wish or desire. For example, 'I have to lose 30kg'.

- Setting unrealistic standards.

- Inability to maintain these standards.

- Feelings of failure and inadequacy again.

- Bingeing.

- Negative self-esteem.

Positive long-term response:

- Set manageable short-term goals.

- Set realistic eating and exercise standards – get some help.

- Gradually improve over time, but take the time to develop good habits.

- Reward yourself along the way.

- Understand that just because it happened in the past doesn't mean it will happen in the present or future.

- Have faith and believe in yourself – you can achieve anything you want.

All or Nothing – Obsessive/Compulsive Personality

Common emotional reaction(s):

- 'If I can't maintain this strict diet, I'm a failure.'

- Either totally strict in every way or out of control.

Positive long-term response:

- Understand that no one can maintain such a strict existence.

- Set yourself more manageable and maintainable goals.

- Enjoy your eating and include some indulgences – it's okay.

- If you do have a meal you would prefer not to have, then don't feel guilty. Get back on track the next meal you have.

- Be consistent NOT unrealistic.

Mid-afternoon and Evening Craving and Bingeing

Common emotional reaction(s):

- 'If I don't get some chocolate quickly I will pass out!'

- Overeating at the time of the day when your body least needs large quantities of food.

Positive long-term response:

- Understand that your cravings are largely due to low blood sugar levels.

- Eat more food in the morning and during the day to maintain blood sugar levels at an appropriate level.

- Make a considered decision to eat based on logic, not emotion or desperation.

Unrealistic Body Image

Due to media portrayal of what 'is normal'.

Common emotional reaction(s):

- Feelings of inadequacy.

- Unrealistic view of self.

- Attempts to lose weight quickly.

- Partake in quick weight-loss scams and diets.

- The possible development of eating disorders.

Positive long-term response:

- Understand that media-imposed standards are not the norm.

- Accept your body shape and address only the things you can change.

- Be realistic in your approach – think long-term.

Height/Weight Charts

Common emotional reaction:

- 'I weigh too much and have to lose weight.'

Positive long-term response:

- Understand the height-weight relationship and that every body is different.

- There is no one chart that can possibly cater for every person.

- Get some objective and professional input and advice.

I hope I been able to clarify a few things in this chapter. While reading this if you have said to yourself 'That's me', then I urge you to address these issues. It is very difficult to move forward physically if you have issues emotionally and psychologically.

You are the most important person in the world. I want you to stand up, find a private place, hug yourself and say out aloud 'I love me'. Do this every day and really mean it.

I promise myself:
To think only of the best
To work only for the best
And expect only the best

I promise myself:
To talk health, happiness and prosperity to every person I meet

I promise myself:
To wear a cheerful countenance at all times
And give every living creature I meet a smile

I promise:
To be just as enthusiastic about the success of others as I am about my own

I promise myself:
To look at the positive side of everything and make my optimism come true

I promise myself:
To make all my friends feel that there is a special something in them
To forget the mistakes of the past and press on to the greater achievements of the future

I promise myself:
To give so much time to the improvement of myself that I have no time to criticize others

I promise myself:
To be too large for worry, too noble for anger, too strong for fear and too happy to permit the presence of trouble

Because:
My attitude is my life

Supporting References

Cardwell, G., *Diet Addiction* (1994), Wellness Australia.

Jampolsky, Dr G.G., *Forgiveness – The Greatest Healer of All* (1999), Beyond Words Publishing Inc, NY.

14
Coping With Eating Out and Other Social Events

One of the most enjoyable aspects of life is spending quality time with good friends and family. It is unavoidable that for the most part these social occasions will be organised around eating and drinking. Christmas feasts, birthday cakes, wedding receptions, dinners with friends, lunches with family, out for drinks, coffee and cake . . . where does it end?

It is an unfortunate reality that most people associate eating out with 'bad' or 'unhealthy' food and too much alcohol. They go to extraordinary lengths to avoid these situations and consequently miss out or experience stress leading up to social outings. Not only are they trying to avoid foods that will 'make them fat', but also the reactions and negative influences of others in the social circle.

Let me just say at this point that it is quite possible to eat out with minimal damage to your body or your progress. If eating out is an occasional thing then sometimes it is okay to eat what you want and enjoy it.

Okay, let's have a look at some of the things you can do to make your social eating a relatively healthy, less stressful and more enjoyable experience.

General Considerations

1 Eat at as normal a time as possible to minimise hunger.

2 Make sure you eat regularly and well during the day leading up to the social event.

3 Don't decrease your food intake during the day to 'have plenty of room and get your money's worth'.

4 Have something to eat before you go out if you are:
   a. Hungry
   b. Likely to be eating later than normal
   c. Dining at a location where you are unsure of the quality of the food.

5 Choose restaurants that can and will accommodate your needs.

6 Ensure friends and family understand your eating require-ments in advance to avoid any awkward situations.

7 Try to break the associations between events and food, for example:
   a. Movies and choc tops, lollies and popcorn
   b. Football and pies, chips and beer.

8 Establish new associations such as:
   a. Movies and snuggling!
   b. Football and bonding with friends and harrassing the umpires!

At the Venue

1 Seat yourself away from the dessert display. Looking at delicious cakes when you are hungry is not a good idea.

2 Ask for water as soon as you are seated. It's a good move to get water in your hand and in your mouth as soon as possible, particularly if you are planning to drink alcohol.

3 Avoid eating a lot of bread before the meal – it's too easy to overeat, especially if you are hungry.

4 At dinner parties:
   a. Don't sit near the food and nibbles table.
   b. Don't arrive hungry – eat before leaving home.
   c. Offer to bring your own dish – then there will be at least one meal you know you can eat.

Ordering

When looking at the menu, don't look at the desserts first.

Read the menu and understand the description of the meals. Here are some common words and their meanings:

Deluxe – large portion size
Sautéed – can mean fried
Alfredo – creamy white sauce
Crumbed – usually fried
Au gratin – coated in cheese
Crispy – crumbed and fried
Golden brown – crumbed and fried

Ask questions about the meals if you're unsure. For example, how the food is cooked, how is it served, what the sauce is.

Order before others at the table to avoid being influenced by their choices.

Ask for the meal to be changed to suit your requirements. Be assertive and don't worry about what others think or say. Any good restaurant will be happy to vary an order for you. If they refuse to deviate from the menu, eat what you can, then don't go back.

Some common requests that I make whenever I eat out:

- Salad with dressing on the side

- Fish or steak without the sauce or with the sauce on the side

- Extra vegetables or salad instead of chips or potatoes

- Grilled not fried

- Pasta with a tomato base instead of cream, and no cheese.

These are just some adjustments you can request. If you don't feel comfortable asking for these changes you need to decide whether to eat your meal as it comes or eat what you can on the plate then see if anyone else wants what you have left.

If the portion sizes are too large:

- Order an entrée as main course

- Order a soup or salad

- Request a half serve

- Share your meal

- Leave what you can't eat – don't feel like you have to eat it all.

Avoid smorgasbord, but if you can't then don't over do it.

Try to keep your meals and ordering as simple as possible. The more involved the meal, the more chance it will contain ingredients of lesser nutritional quality.

Eating

1 Slow down your eating so that the feeling of fullness will settle in before you've been able to overeat. It takes about 20 minutes for the brain to realise you are full.

2 Take a break between courses.

3 Make sure you wait at least 20 minutes after the main course before deciding whether you really need dessert.

4 When you've finished eating, have the dishes cleared fast to avoid picking.

5 Dessert (if necessary):
  a. Fresh fruit
  b. Share or half serve
  c. If it is only occasional, eat it and enjoy it.

6 Drinks:
  a. Lots of water
  b. Use soda as a mixer rather than soft drink
  c. Dilute your drinks, e.g. champagne and OJ, half shots of spirits
  d. Moderation
  e. Herbal tea and skim milk coffee.

The Festive Season

End-of-Year Function Strategies

- It is important to consider all the points already mentioned, but at this time of the year there are likely to be numerous functions over a short period of time.

- At all times, avoid turning up to functions hungry, especially if the food is the catered fried 'nibble' variety. A few little nibbles won't kill you, but overeating function food is a poor nutritional choice.

- Choose dips with carrots, celery etc. and non-fried options where possible.

- If attending numerous functions, decide to indulge at one of them and employ the strategies at the others.

- Be assertive – don't be forced to eat food or drink in quantities that you don't want to.

- Maintain or increase your exercise regime over this period. Don't use social functions as an excuse not to exercise – this will compound the negative health effect.

Christmas Day Strategies

- Do some exercise in the morning, and eat a normal breakfast and snack leading up to lunch to avoid low blood sugar levels and excessive hunger.

- Don't overfill your plate, and eat slowly.

- Don't eat everything served if you become full before finishing.

- Sit and digest food for 20 minutes before deciding if you really want seconds.

- Select BBQs, lean meat, seafood and salads. Avoid sauces high in fat or sugar such as gravy, mint sauce, cranberry sauce.

- Enjoy a small serving of pudding.

- Fresh fruit is a good way to finish the meal and cleanse the system.

- Arrange a cricket game or other active game after lunch rather sleeping on the couch.

- Continue the remainder of the day as usual with a light dinner.

- Have a large lunch or dinner but not both.

- Indulge if you wish but aim to exercise the next day.

- Be careful on the days following Christmas. It is very easy to fall into the trap of overeating festive food for a week instead of just one day.

- Focus on how much work it will take to get back to your pre-Christmas shape if you celebrate for too long.

Remember, you can choose one of two healthy options when it comes to enjoying any social event that you will be attending:

1 Decide to indulge yourself and enjoy it, because it only happens every now and again. If this is the case don't beat yourself up and feel guilty for days afterwards.

2 Take steps (as outlined) to ensure your meal is as healthy as possible, without worrying about what everyone else says or thinks.

Both options raise issues that need to be dealt with effectively and without extra stress.

Deciding to indulge yourself raises the issue of indulging without feeling like you have damaged your progress or let yourself down. This is an area I have spoken about in some detail. Remember you are allowed to reward yourself and you need to enjoy your indulgences in moderation. Balance in life is a very healthy thing, so if you can learn to value yourself and realise that it is not a weakness to eat something you enjoy even when you don't think you should, you will live a happier and healthier life.

Taking positive action to eat a certain way, particularly in social situations, will always raise issues that involve other people. Peer group pressure is a very strong influence and you need to understand that many people, no matter what their relationship with you, will not be as supportive as you would like them to be. The reason for this is because, as you get into better shape, it affects the way they feel about themselves. Have you noticed that when you are trying to eat well people will regularly try to pressure you into eating chocolate, cake or some other indulgence? If they see you eating these foods they will not feel guilty about eating. People will often say or do things from a selfish standpoint, even though they may like to be seen as helping you. Be wary.

It is very important that you associate with positive and supportive people or your life will be difficult and you will end up either avoiding social situations or giving up your 'you' plan altogether. Neither of these alternatives is ideal.

Make sure you communicate your eating requirements to your friends and family in advance to avoid uncomfortable situations. My friends know me well enough now to tell me what they are preparing in advance to make sure I will eat it. Yes they joke about it a bit, but I am comfortable with my lifestyle and very happy with how I feel and look as a result of the way I eat.

Many of my clients will justify making poor food choices at dinner parties because they don't want to offend the cook. I say, 'Offend the cook'! Only kidding. But be quite clear on this point: your eating preferences are not a reflection of the cooking but of your needs. It is vital that you make this point clear to your host.

Relax and enjoy your social activities. Live your life by your rules and no one else's. Life is far too short to spend it stressing about what anyone but you thinks.

15
Implementation

I have given you a lot of information to this point. Do you feel comfortable with it? Can you see yourself living the life I suggest? Do you feel able to put your new knowledge into positive, life-changing action?

It is very easy to go to a seminar or read a book and be given a lot of information that sounds good. But information means nothing if it is not acted upon.

This is the stage we are at right now. You have the tools now to change your life for the better. No one can do it but you.

Let me help you take this step, the hardest but by far the most rewarding. I will suggest a plan that you can follow to take this theory and make it reality. The rest is up to you.

This plan is specifically referring to food and eating, but can be used for any other area of your life.

10 Steps to Change Your Life Forever

These steps are progressive. You can't move to the next step until you have **honestly and completely** satisfied the previous step.

Step One

You have already taken the first crucial step. That is, you have realised a need or desire to change. You have bought or borrowed and read this book and probably other books to help motivate you. You consequently have the insight and information necessary to move forward. If this is not the case then you need to either re-read this book or go to some other source to get the information and motivation you require.

Step Two

Make a decision to take action, but don't make this decision lightly.

You need to make this decision for the right reasons: because you want to change for **you** and not because someone else said you should or you think that is what is expected of you. Understand that, in taking this step, you are committing yourself to a course of action that you must maintain. You won't always feel motivated and you may be tempted back to old habits, but you must stick to the new path and persist until it becomes a routine.

Allow yourself the time to create long-term change. Understand that it won't happen quickly, not if you want it to last forever.

If you can accept these conditions then you are ready to move on to Step Three.

Step Three

Involve someone else in the process.

Understand the significance of the step you are taking and its effect on the rest of your life. If you don't feel like you can handle it alone then I suggest you don't even try. Find someone you feel you can trust and let them help and guide you through this crucial stage.

You are responsible for your outcome. Don't blame others if you don't achieve the results you desire.

If you feel you can do it alone then go for it, but don't hesitate to get a professional involved to ensure that you make this your final and successful attempt at creating the person you have always wanted to be.

Step Four

Make a list of your significant food and eating issues and ideas about good nutrition. Your list could include:

- How I feel about myself.

- How I feel about food and eating.

- How I feel about losing weight and dieting.

- My organisation of food.

- Eating breakfast.

- Eating regularly (every 2 to 2½ hours).

- Eating a small dinner.

- Cravings and emotional eating.

- Using the Glycemic Index for controlling blood sugar levels.

- Natural versus processed foods.

- Eating a balance of all foods.

- Shopping and reading labels.

- Indulgences.

- Eating and exercise.

Next to each point on your list, put either a 'smiling face' or a 'tick'. The 'smiling face' refers to areas you are in control of and the 'tick' refers to areas that require some attention. You will now have two lists. The 'tick' list is the one you need to deal with.

Once you have your 'tick' list move to Step Five.

Step Five

Don't try to change the whole 'tick' list at once. Your list may have anywhere from one to 15 items on it. Choose only one or two or as many as you can realistically deal with at any one time. Don't set standards that are too high, otherwise you will fail.

When you have decided upon your first area, move to Step Six.

Step Six

I strongly recommend that you involve someone else in this step (see Step Three).

Set short, medium and long-term goals and actions. Make sure the goals are S.M.A.R.T.

- S – Specific to you, your needs and your desire to improve progressively.

- M – Measurable, i.e. you know when a goal has been achieved.

- A – Ambitious but achievable.

- R – Realistic for you.

- T – Time frame for achievement.

Of the items on your 'tick' list, some will be easier to deal with than others. Let's have a look at some examples.

Example One – 'I need to eat breakfast every day.'

- Short-term goal – To eat a small piece of fruit, one piece of toast or a small bowl of cereal within 30 minutes of getting up, at least three days per week by the end of one month.

- Medium-term goal – To eat a substantial breakfast (two pieces of rye toast with tomato and avocado or a bowl of cereal with fruit and yoghurt) within 30 minutes of getting up, at least five days per week by the end of three months.

- Long-term goal – To eat a high GI piece of fruit within 10 minutes and a substantial natural low GI breakfast within 30 minutes of getting up every day by the end of six months.

In each of the above examples the S.M.A.R.T. principle was applied.

Example Two – 'I need to feel better about myself.'

- Short-term goal – Make an appointment with a psychologist, positive friend or mentor to discuss these feelings, by the end of the week.

- Medium and long-term goals – To be discussed, organised and implemented with help from the above person.

Example Three – 'I need to stop the sugar cravings and binge eating that starts at 4pm and lasts all night.'

- Short-term goal – To keep an accurate food diary, outlining all food and drink consumed, the times of the day, activities, energy levels and emotional states each day for two weeks. This is to create an awareness and understanding of the way you feel and the associations with eating.

- Medium-term goal – To learn from information gathered from the food diary. To eat at least three low GI balanced meals/snacks before 4pm each day by the end of two months.

- Long-term goal – To eat breakfast (as above) and a balanced and natural low GI snack or meal every two hours until 4pm each day by the end of four months.

Once you have set your short, medium and long-term goals for each area move to Step Seven.

Step Seven

Follow your plan consistently.

Your goals may be to lose fat, have more energy or be healthier. By acting consistently you will reach these goals without obsessing about them. Accept that there will be times when, for whatever reason, you will be unable to follow your plan to the letter. You just need to be able to get back on the plan as soon as possible, and stay positive at all times.

Commit yourself regardless of how you are feeling, your emotional state day to day, your conditioning or what other people around you are saying – PERSIST.

Follow your plan for the set time period and then move to Step Eight.

Step Eight

Review your progress regularly and modify your goals and actions if necessary.

This is a crucial step. It is imperative that you stop and reflect on your progress every so often. This may happen every week, every two weeks, every month or every three months. Reviews will become less frequent as time goes on and routines become established.

During each review session ask yourself the following questions:

- Can I maintain this change in lifestyle?

- Am I enjoying this new routine?

- Have I noticed a positive difference?

- Am I changing my attitudes and thinking?

- Are the time frames I have set realistic?

If the answer to any of the above questions was not what you would have liked, it is okay. It doesn't mean you are a failure, it simply means that you need to devise a slightly different path and modify your goals to achieve your desired outcome. There are many ways to achieve the same outcome, and you may need to explore several of them until you find your most preferred path. If you need to give yourself a bit more time, then do it. If you need to change some of the foods you first decided upon, then do that too. If your priorities change, make the appropriate modifications.

There are no failures, only experiences to be learnt from. Learn then move on. **Always stay positive**. Keep reviewing and modifying (if needed) until you have taken your goal and established it as a new behaviour.

Once you have achieved this with each of your chosen areas, move to Step Nine.

Step Nine

Transfer the newly established routines from the 'tick' list to the 'smiling face' list and then go back to Step Five and choose your next areas for attention. Follow the plan from Step Five through to this point.

Once you have completed the entire 'tick' list and have moved all items to the 'smiling face' list move to Step Ten.

Step Ten

Enjoy your new life and all the benefits it provides.

Part 2

Recipes

Recipes

It is time to cook up a storm!

I have included a selection of recipes from various sources. The recipes include the following:

1   Breakfasts

2   Soups

3   Salads

4   Sides and accompaniments

5   Light meals

6   Main meals

7   Snacks and desserts

All recipes have been modified to ensure they:

* Taste great

* Are low GI

* Are very low in saturated fats and trans-fatty acids

- Are low in overall fat, but do include some healthy fats

- Include fresh, natural and wholegrain ingredients

- Are free from processed and artificial ingredients

- Are easy to prepare.

Bear in mind that the main aim of this book is to help you become the person you have always wanted to be. That means not having to rely on anyone but yourself and knowing and understanding what is required to live a long, healthy and happy life. So why am I saying this now? Because while I am supplying you with these recipes, I want you to know that it is pretty easy to modify and manipulate any recipe you have to one that fulfils the above criteria. All you need to know is what simple substitutions can be made to transform your favourite recipe. Great tasting, healthy and creative cooking, as with everything, is in your hands.

Here is an example. Let's say you are a curry lover and you have found the following recipe for a prawn curry.

Prawn Curry

Serves 6
2 tbsp vegetable oil
2 onions thinly sliced
1 green capsicum, seeded and sliced
500g pumpkin peeled and diced
½ cup curry paste
1 tbsp sugar
1kg green prawns, peeled and de-veined
425g can chopped tomatoes
140ml coconut milk
½ cup chopped coriander
1 cup uncooked white rice

There are a few changes I would make to the ingredients before I attempted to cook this:

1 Either replace the vegetable oil with extra virgin olive oil (half the amount listed) or use water or stock to sauté the onions and capsicum.

2 Replace the high GI pumpkin with low GI sweet potato.

3 Instead of curry paste, unless you can find a good one without a lot of sugars, bad fats or artificial additives, use curry powder and other herbs and spices such as coriander and cumin.

4 Why does it need sugar? Leave it out.

5 Make sure that the can of chopped tomatoes is without added sugar or salt.

6 Instead of coconut milk, stir through natural yoghurt just before serving.

7 Replace the white rice with a basmati rice or a white or brown long grain rice.

You will still end up with a delicious meal, but one that is much better for you. Can you see how easy it is? Just to make sure, here is another quick example, a recipe for home-made pizza.

Home-Made Pizza

1 pre-prepared pizza base
1 small container pizza sauce
1 cup grated mozzarella cheese
200g sliced salami
Onion, capsicum, mushroom etc. sliced

I am sure you can see what we need to do with this recipe.

1   Instead of the pre-prepared base, use pita bread (prefer-
    ably rye if you can get it).

2   The pizza sauce is likely to contain sugar and salt. Use a
    tomato paste with no added salt or sugar and add your
    own herbs and spices for flavour.

3   Use a half serve of cheese, low-fat cheese, cottage cheese
    or no cheese, whatever your preference.

4   Avoid the salami – replace it with lean 'off the bone' ham,
    lean chicken or seafood.

5   Load it up with lots of vegetables.

Do you feel comfortable with making these changes? I want
you to feel totally confident that, regardless of the recipe, you
can modify it to suit your needs.

Here is a list of ingredients and simple substitutions to
make when 'cooking up a storm' to ensure maximum taste,
health and energy:

1   An abundance of fresh fruits and vegetables.

2   Rye, wholegrain, soy and linseed, sourdough rye and pita
    breads instead of highly refined white and wholemeal

bread. Use the squeeze test: if it is light and fluffy put it back on the shelf.

3 Basmati or long grain rice instead of standard white or jasmine.

4 Sweet potato instead of potato and pumpkin.

5 Wholegrain and fresh pastas.

6 Grains other than wheat, e.g. oats, buckwheat, bulgur (burghul), oat bran and barley.

7 Rye or chickpea flour instead of white.

8 Replace some meat with beans, soy beans, chickpeas, lentils, nuts and tofu.

9 Fresh and lean meats.

10 Fish and seafood.

11 Make your own sauces, marinades and dressings:
   • Salt-reduced tamari (soy sauce)
   • Tomato paste or fresh crushed tomatoes
   • Extra virgin olive oil
   • Red wine and balsamic vinegar
   • Herbs and spices
   • Mustard (free from added sugar)
   • Lemon juice
   • Fresh ginger and garlic
   • Stock cubes or prepared stocks
   • Yellow box or other low GI honey

12 When sweetening foods use sugar in moderation. Preferably use puréed fruit, natural fruit juice, dried fruit or a low GI honey. Some sugar may be used in moderation.

Avoid artificial sweeteners even though they have fewer calories.

13 Use low-fat milks and natural yoghurts (ideally low-fat and naturally sweetened). Avoid creams.

14 Use low-fat cheeses: cottage, ricotta, fetta.

15 Use eggs; one yolk per six whites is enough to give you a complete protein.

Remember that every now and then if you find a recipe that you really like, leave the recipe as it is, cook it and enjoy it. Moderation is the key.

I hope you enjoy the following recipes.

BREAKFAST

VANILLA BEAN MUESLI (GRANOLA) (WHEAT-FREE)

1kg rolled oats
500g amaranth
50g sunflower seeds
50g pumpkin seeds
100g dried apricots, chopped
100g sultanas
100g dried apple, chopped
zest of 1 orange
1 vanilla bean split and centre removed

- Combine rolled oats, amaranth and seeds in a large bowl and mix thoroughly.
- Add chopped apricots, apples and sultanas and mix until distributed evenly.
- Add orange zest and centre of vanilla bean and mix through.
- Store in airtight container.

Serving suggestions

- ½ cup of muesli with ½ cup natural yoghurt, 1 tsp yellow box honey and sliced banana and/or strawberries.
- ½ cup of muesli with ½ cup flavoured yoghurt and ¼ cup fresh berries.
- ½ cup of muesli with low fat milk and stewed apple.
- Use as a base for Bircher muesli (see next page).

Recipe information
Serves: makes 2kg (4.4lb) muesli
Preparation time: 15 minutes

CAFÉ STYLE BIRCHER MUESLI

1 cup wheat-free muesli (granola) (see previous recipe) or
sugar free natural muesli

½ cup apple juice (100%), no added sugar

½ cup natural or natural fruit yoghurt (low fat)

1 fresh apple, grated or ½ cup unsweetened canned chopped
apple

½ cup frozen or fresh berries

- Combine muesli with apple juice.
- Soak overnight.
- Combine soaked muesli with fresh apple, berries and
  yoghurt, just before serving.

Serving suggestions

- Serve 1 cup of combined mix in large cereal bowls.
- Garnish with fresh strawberries.

Recipe information
Serves: approx 4
Preparation time: 5–10 minutes (plus overnight soaking)

PERFECT PORRIDGE

1 cup rolled oats
1 tbsp sultanas
1 tsp cinnamon
1 tsp linseeds
1 tbsp protein powder (optional)
1½ cups water

- Combine oats, sultanas, cinnamon and linseeds. Mix thoroughly.
- Add water and soak overnight.
- For high protein porridge add protein powder plus ½ cup extra water to soaked mix.

Cooking methods

- Combine dry ingredients with 1½ cups boiling water.
- Microwave on high for 3 minutes or cook on stove for 5 minutes, add extra water as required.

Serving suggestions

- Serve 1 cup with yellow box honey and half a sliced banana.
- Serve 1 cup with ½ cup stewed fruit such as apple or rhubarb or poached pears.

Recipe information
Serves: 2
Preparation time: 5 minutes (plus overnight soaking)
Cooking time: 3 minutes

BUCKWHEAT PANCAKES

½ cup ground almonds
½ cup buckwheat flour
¾ cup water
OR
1 cup buckwheat flour
1 cup water
1 tbsp arrowroot

- Blend all ingredients thoroughly until smooth.
- Heat non-stick pan with a small amount of olive oil.
- Pour desired amount of mixture into pan and cook until the edges of the pancakes begin to lift from the pan.
- Turn pancake and briefly cook other side.

Serving suggestions

- Serve warm with unsweetened fruit jam and sliced strawberries.
- Serve warm with yellow box honey, cinnamon and banana.

Recipe information
Serves: 5–8 pancakes (depending on size)
Preparation time: 5–10 minutes
Cooking time: 5 minutes

SUPER SMOOTHIES

Base Ingredients

3 tbsp sugar free, low fat yoghurt

½ cup of 100% fruit juice (apple, grapefruit, pear)

1 tsp flaxseed oil

1 tsp yellow box honey (optional)

2 tbsp unflavoured/vanilla protein powder (optional)

Mix base ingredients in a blender with any of the following (or make up your own).

Banana and Pecan (or LSA: crushed linseeds, sunflower seeds and almonds)

- 1 frozen ripe banana
- 6 pecans (or 1 tbsp LSA)

Summer Berries

- 1 cup frozen mixed berries (strawberries, blueberries, raspberries, blackberries)

Vanilla and Strawberry

- ½ vanilla bean
- 1 cup fresh strawberries

Banana and Blueberry

- ½ frozen banana
- ½ cup frozen/fresh blueberries

Recipe information

Serves: 1

Preparation time: 5 minutes

SOUPS

TOMATO AND BASIL SOUP OR SAUCE

1 large onion
2 × 410g (14 oz) cans of diced tomatoes
½ cup tomato paste
1 bunch of basil
2 cloves garlic
2 cups vegetable stock

Soup

- Chop onions and add to a heated pan with garlic, sauté until soft.
- Add canned tomatoes and vegetable stock.
- Strip basil leaves and julienne, set aside.
- When tomatoes come to the boil reduce heat and simmer for 30 minutes.
- Add tomato paste and basil leaves, salt and pepper to taste and simmer for 5–7 minutes.
- Re-adjust seasoning and serve.

Sauce

- Leave out vegetable stock and follow steps above.
- Serve with fresh pasta or grilled meats.

Variation

- Add baby spinach with basil and tomato paste to make spinach, basil and tomato soup.

> ***Recipe information***
> Serves: 4
> Preparation time: 10 minutes
> Cooking time: 50 minutes

CURRIED BEAN AND MUSHROOM SOUP

½ cup of dried red kidney beans (or equivalent canned)
½ cup of dried black-eyed beans (or equivalent canned)
1 small leek, sliced thinly
1 small carrot, julienned
125g (4.4 oz) baby mushrooms, sliced
1 tsp curry powder
410g (14 oz) can crushed tomatoes
3 cups vegetable stock
1 tsp fresh parsley

- Place dried beans in a large bowl, cover with boiling water, stand for 1 hour and then drain.
- Cook dried beans in lots of boiling water for about 25 minutes or until tender, drain.
- Sauté leeks in a little vegetable stock for about 4–5 minutes or until leeks are soft.
- Add carrots, mushroom and curry powder.
- Stir over medium heat for 1–2 minutes.
- Stir in beans, undrained crushed tomatoes and remaining stock.
- Bring to the boil, reduce heat, cover and simmer for about 25 minutes.
- Stir in parsley.

Recipe information
Serves: 6
Preparation time: 20 minutes
Cooking time: 60 minutes

ROASTED RED PEPPER (BELL PEPPER) SOUP OR PASTA SAUCE

10 red capsicums (bell peppers)
350g (12 oz) plum tomatoes
1 litre (2 pints) vegetable stock
Pinch sea salt and cayenne pepper

- Roast whole capsicums on baking tray in 200°C (400°F) oven for 30 minutes until skin bubbles and blackens.
- Place in a plastic bag or covered bowl for 10–20 minutes.
- Peel and deseed capsicums and keep juices.
- Remove skin from tomatoes.
- Blend capsicum flesh and juice and peeled tomatoes in food processor.
- Season with sea salt and cayenne pepper.

Soup

Add vegetable stock to blended sauce and bring to the boil.
Reduce heat and simmer for a few minutes before serving.

Pasta Sauce

Toss blended sauce with cooked fresh pasta.
Garnish with fresh basil and serve.

Protein variations

- Add cubed firm tofu to soup, simmer and serve.
- Add steamed broccoli and cooked chicken to pasta sauce and toss with pasta.
- Add drained tuna (in spring water) and sliced blanched zucchini to pasta sauce and toss with pasta.

Recipe information

Serves: 4

Preparation time: 20 minutes

Cooking time: 40 minutes

SWEET POTATO AND WALNUT SOUP

1 medium onion
1 clove of garlic, crushed (minced)
300g (10.6 oz) sweet potato, peeled and cut into small
  chunks
1½ cups of vegetable stock
2 tsp tomato paste
2 tbsp chopped walnuts

- Sauté onion and garlic in a small amount of vegetable stock for 1–2 minutes over a medium heat.
- Add the sweet potato, remaining stock, tomato paste and walnuts and bring to the boil.
- Reduce the heat, cover and simmer for about 30 minutes.
- Allow to cool then blend the sweet potato mixture until smooth.
- Add extra stock or water to achieve desired consistency.
- Reheat before serving and sprinkle with chopped walnuts.

Recipe information
Serves: 4
Preparation time: 110 minutes
Cooking time: 40 minutes

SWEET POTATO AND LENTIL SOUP

1 onion

1 medium sweet potato, chopped

1 cup red lentils

1 litre (2.2 pints) vegetable stock

- Sauté onion in a little stock.
- Add remaining ingredients.
- Bring to the boil, reduce heat, cover and simmer for about 20 minutes.
- Blend in batches until smooth.
- Add extra stock or water to achieve desired consistency.
- Reheat before serving.
- Serve with a swirl of natural yoghurt (if desired).

Recipe information

Serves: 4

Preparation time: 10 minutes

Cooking time: 30 minutes

CHICKEN AND SWEETCORN SOUP

6 cups chicken stock

2–3 cups water

2 chicken breast fillets, trimmed

5 shallots (green onions), thinly sliced

1 clove garlic, crushed (minced)

3 corn cobs, kernels removed

2 tbsp Chinese cooking wine

1½ tbsp tamari

coriander (cilantro) for garnish

- Bring water and stock to boil in large saucepan.
- Reduce heat, add chicken and simmer for 6 minutes.
- Remove chicken from stock, cool and then shred.
- Add shallots, garlic, corn kernels, wine and tamari to stock.
- Simmer for 5 minutes and then remove from heat.
- Cool slightly then process half the soup in blender.
- Return processed soup to remaining stock, add chicken and simmer until heated through.
- Serve and sprinkle with coriander.

Recipe information

Serves: 4

Preparation time: 15 minutes

SALADS

TABOULI

250g (8.8 oz) dry bulgur wheat
4 large tomatoes, finely chopped
1 green capsicum (bell pepper), finely chopped
½ cucumber, finely chopped
1 clove garlic, crushed (minced)
1 red onion, finely chopped
juice of 2 lemons
1 cup chopped flat leaf parsley
2–3 tbsp chopped mint
salt and pepper

- Put bulgur wheat in a bowl.
- Add all ingredients and season with salt and pepper.
- Cover and refrigerate for 12 hours.

Serving suggestions

- Side dish to barbecued meats.
- Serve with chicken burgers (see recipe).
- Serve with falafels and hommus dip.
- Use in sandwiches, wraps and burgers.

Recipe information
Serves: 6–8
Preparation time: 20 minutes (plus 12 hours in fridge)

CANNELLINI BEAN SALAD

2 × 400g (14 oz) cans cannellini beans (no added sugar)
1 Spanish onion, finely chopped
3 Roma tomatoes, finely chopped
2 tsp ground cumin seeds
½ cup fresh herbs, chopped (parsley, chives, basil)

- Drain beans, add to large bowl.
- Add onion, tomato and cumin and mix well.
- Toss through herbs.

Serving suggestions

- As a side dish to barbecued fish, chicken, lamb or steak.
- Add shredded chicken or tuna for a light lunch.

Recipe information
Serves: 4
Preparation time: 10 minutes

ROAST VEGIE SALAD

1 large Spanish onion
1 large sweet potato
1 large zucchini
1 large eggplant
750g (1.6 lb) button mushrooms
400g tin artichokes in brine
2 tbsp tomato paste
2 tbsp balsamic vinegar
chopped flat leaf parsley
cos lettuce to serve

- Preheat oven to 200°C (400°F).
- Cut all vegetables into 1cm (½ inch) pieces, leaving the artichokes whole.
- Fry artichokes on hot grill until brown, leave to cool.
- Combine the tomato paste with the balsamic vinegar.
- Coat all the vegetables except artichokes with tomato paste mix.
- Spread vegetables over roasting tray and bake in oven for 30 minutes or until the potato is soft.
- Leave to cool.
- Toss through parsley.
- Place a bed of cos lettuce in large serving bowl.
- Fill up with roasted vegetables and add sliced artichokes on top.

Protein variation

- Add shredded roast chicken or tuna to cold vegetable mix.

Recipe information
Serves: 8
Preparation time: 20 minutes
Cooking time: 30 minutes

ROCKET, TUNA AND HARICOT BEAN SALAD

4 tomatoes, skinned, deseeded and roughly chopped
125g (4.4 oz) rocket
400g (14 oz) can haricot beans, drained
200g (7 oz) can tuna in spring water, drained
1 red onion, chopped
400g (4.4 oz) artichoke hearts in brine, sliced
2 celery sticks (stalks) with inner leaves, chopped
1 tbsp pitted black olives
4 tbsp lemon juice
1 tbsp red wine vinegar
¼ tsp crushed (minced) dried chilli
handful of flat leaf parsley, roughly chopped
salt and pepper

- Put tomatoes in a large salad bowl with the rocket.
- Stir in the beans and tuna, roughly breaking the tuna into large chunks.
- Stir in the red onion.
- Add the artichoke hearts, the celery, olives, lemon juice, vinegar, chilli and parsley.
- Season with salt and pepper to taste.
- Mix all the ingredients together well and allow to stand for 30 minutes for the flavours to mingle.
- Serve the salad at room temperature.

Recipe information
Serves: 4
Preparation time: 15 minutes (plus 30 minutes resting
time)

LAYERED NIÇOISE SALAD

1 400g (14 oz) can tuna in spring water
4 hard boiled eggs
200g (7 oz) green beans, blanched
12 olives, finely sliced
1 Spanish onion, chopped finely
4 Roma tomatoes
2 cooked corn cobs, kernels removed
salt and pepper

- Slice Roma tomatoes in half and roast in a hot oven for 15 minutes. Allow to cool.
- Drain tuna and combine with Spanish onion, corn and olives and season with salt and pepper.
- Serve in layers starting with blanched beans, roast tomatoes, tuna mix and top with sliced boiled eggs.

Recipe information
Serves: 4
Preparation time: 20 minutes
Cooking time: 15 minutes

GREEK STYLE SALAD

1 cos lettuce
250g (8.8 oz) cherry tomatoes
½ continental cucumber
150g (5.3 oz) low fat fetta cheese
1 Spanish onion
1 red capsicum (bell pepper)

- Roast red capsicum in hot oven for 20 minutes.
- Place in plastic bag and leave for 10 minutes.
- Remove skin and seeds and cut into thin strips.
- Save juice for dressing.
- Wash lettuce well and spin dry.
- Chop tomatoes in halves, cucumber and fetta into bite size pieces and onion into thin half rings.
- Combine all ingredients in a large bowl.
- Dress with salad dressing (see below).
- Garnish with roast capsicum strips.

Sally's Salad dressing

½ cup of roasted capsicum juice (see above)
1 tbsp olive oil
1 tbsp balsamic vinegar

- Combine ingredients in a small bowl.
- Whisk until well combined.

Recipe information
Serves: 6
Preparation time: 25 minutes
Cooking time: 20 minutes

SIDES AND ACCOMPANIMENTS

HOME-MADE HOMMUS

½ cup dry chickpeas (garbanzo beans) or 400g (14 oz) can
½ cup water
1 tbsp lemon juice
1 tsp olive oil
1 clove crushed garlic (minced)
1 tbsp tamari

- Soak chickpeas overnight, drain and cover with fresh water.
- Cook until tender and drain.
- Add water and other ingredients gradually.
- Blend well.
- Store in airtight container in fridge.

Serving suggestions

- Serve as a dip with celery, carrot, cucumber, broccoli and/or mushrooms.
- Serve with warm rye pita bread.
- Use as a spread for sandwiches.

Recipe information
Preparation time: 10 minutes
Cooking time: 30 minutes (plus overnight soaking)

TOMATO AND CAPSICUM (BELL PEPPER) SALSA

8 vine ripened tomatoes
2 red capsicums (bell peppers)
8 basil leaves, torn
1 tbsp red wine vinegar
1 tsp extra virgin olive oil

- Cut each tomato into 8 wedges and place in a greased, shallow oven-proof dish (pan) and bake for 30–40 minutes at 200°C (400°F).
- Roast whole capsicums in oven until blackened.
- Place capsicums in a bowl and cover tightly with plastic wrap (or place in a plastic bag). Leave for 10 minutes, then peel off the skin and remove seeds. Slice finely.
- Remove tomatoes from oven.
- Combine tomatoes with capsicum and basil.
- Whisk together the vinegar and oil, pour over the tomato mixture and gently toss.
- Season with salt and pepper to taste.
- Serve as a dip or as a tasty sauce for chicken, turkey or fish.

Recipe information
Preparation time: 15–20 minutes
Cooking time: 30–40 minutes

GRILLED ASPARAGUS WITH OLIVE OIL AND SEA SALT

1kg fresh asparagus, trimmed
2 tbsp extra virgin olive oil
sea salt

- Place asparagus on a grill pan that is smoking hot.
- Allow to char on both sides (by then asparagus should be cooked).
- Serve drizzled with olive oil, and season with sea salt.
- Serve as a side dish to barbecue meat, roasts or other protein dishes.

Variation

- Sprinkle grilled asparagus with sesame seeds.

Recipe information
Serves: 4
Serving size: 8 spears
Preparation time: 5 minutes
Cooking time: 3 minutes

SWEET POTATO MASH

1kg sweet potato
sea salt and cracked pepper

- Peel potatoes and cut into equal size pieces.
- Just cover with water, add salt and boil until tender.
- When cooked, drain and allow to stand for 4 minutes.
- Mash to break down pieces.
- Season with sea salt and cracked black pepper.

Variation

- Use 200g of black pitted olives.
- Blend half (100g) olives in a food processor.
- Roughly chop remaining half (100g).
- Add to the mashed potato.
- Season with cracked pepper (extra salt not required as the olives are salty).

Recipe information
Serves: 6
Preparation time: 10–15 minutes
Cooking time: 5–10 minutes

RATATOULLIE

1 small eggplant, cubed
1 large red pepper
1 green pepper
2 zucchini
2 onions
2 cloves of garlic
1 tsp thyme
500g Roma tomatoes
fresh basil
salt and pepper

- Chop eggplant, peppers and zucchini into 3cm (1.2 inch) chunks.
- Chop onions and tomatoes into wedges.
- Finely chop garlic.
- Combine all the vegetables, garlic, thyme and salt and pepper in an oven-proof casserole dish.
- Bake in a moderate oven (180°C/350°F) for between 30 and 40 minutes.
- Toss through torn basil.

Serving suggestions

- Serve warm as side dish to fish, chicken, lamb or steak.
- Stir through cooked pasta.
- Serve cold as salad.

Recipe information
Serves: 4
Preparation time: 10–15 minutes
Cooking time: 30–40 minutes

LIGHT MEALS

FABULOUS FRIED RICE

2 cups raw basmati or long grain brown rice
1 capsicum (bell pepper)
2 onions
2 cobs corn
100g shitake mushrooms (soaked 30 minutes)
2 eggs
1 bunch baby bok choy
1 tsp ginger
2–3 tbsp tamari
pinch of chilli powder

- Cook rice, rinse with cold water and drain well. Place in the coldest part of the refrigerator allowing the rice to drain as it cools.
- Julienne capsicum, onion, mushrooms, bok choy and ginger.
- Sauté all vegetables and ginger in wok.
- Add chilli.
- Add cooked rice and tamari.
- Lightly beat eggs in small dish.
- Make room in wok to cook egg, keep turning until cooked evenly.
- Stir egg through rice mixture and toss until tamari has coated all rice (add more if required).
- Season with additional tamari to taste.

Variation

- Add 500g of lean ham, shrimps or cooked chicken.

Recipe information
Serves: 4
Preparation time: 20–30 minutes
Cooking time: 10 minutes

DAHL

2½ cups brown lentils

2 medium onions

2 small red chillies (chilli peppers), finely chopped

1 tsp ground cumin

1 tsp ground coriander (cilantro)

½ tsp garam masala

½ tsp ground cardamon

1 tsp ground tumeric

1½ litres (3 pints) vegetable stock

- Place lentils in large bowl, cover with water, stand overnight and then drain.
- Sauté onion, chilli, cumin, coriander, garam masala and cardamon in a small amount of vegetable stock over a medium heat for about 2 minutes.
- Stir in lentils, remaining vegetable stock and tumeric.
- Bring to the boil, reduce heat, simmer uncovered for 50 minutes or until mixture has thickened to your desired consistency.

Serving suggestions

- Use as a side dish to fish, chicken or meat.
- Serve as a meal with basmati or long grain rice and pappadams.
- Can be eaten cold as a dip.

Tip

Pappadams can be cooked in the microwave on high for 15 seconds each.

Recipe information

Serves: 8–10

Preparation time: 10 minutes (plus overnight soaking)

Cooking time: 60 minutes

SALLY'S SPINACH PIE

1 onion

200g (7 oz) lean ham 'off the bone' (without – for vegetarian option)

5 whole eggs

5 egg whites

1 grated zucchini

1 grated carrot

1 bunch English spinach or silver beet, finely chopped

1 tsp nutmeg

salt and pepper

1 tsp baking powder

1 cup wholemeal (whole wheat) self raising flour

2 tomatoes

- Grease large, flat ovenproof pan with a small amount of olive oil.
- Line bottom with greaseproof (wax) paper.
- Preheat oven to 180°C (350°F).
- Cook onion and ham until onion is soft.
- Mix onion and ham with grated carrot, zucchini and spinach in a large bowl.
- Add baking powder and flour to vegetables and mix until well distributed.
- Beat eggs and egg whites until fluffy; add salt, pepper and nutmeg.
- Add eggs to vegetables and fold until combined.
- Pour mixture into pan.
- Slice tomatoes and arrange on top.
- Bake in oven for 40 minutes or until egg is set (test with skewer).
- Serve warm or cold with salad.

Variations

- Omit ham for vegetarian spinach pie.
- Substitute wholemeal (whole wheat) flour with barley or rice flour for wheat free.

Recipe information
Serves: 6
Preparation time: 20 minutes
Cooking time: 40 minutes

SPINACH AND CHICKPEA (GARBANZO BEAN) SLICE

175g (6 oz) spinach leaves
2 tsp extra virgin olive oil
1 small onion, thinly sliced
2 garlic cloves, crushed (minced)
1 tsp ground turmeric
200g (7 oz) canned chickpeas (garbanzo beans), drained
2 whole eggs and 2 extra egg whites
200ml (⅞ cup) skimmed milk
pinch of grated nutmeg
salt and pepper

- Preheat oven to 180°C (350°F).
- Line a shallow oven pan with greaseproof (wax) paper.
- Wash the spinach and place in a large saucepan.
- Heat gently for 3–4 minutes until the spinach wilts.
- Drain, squeeze out the excess liquid and chop finely.
- Heat the oil in a saucepan, add the onion, garlic and turmeric and sauté for 5 minutes.
- Stir in the chickpeas (garbanzo beans) and spinach then remove from the heat – spread mixture over the pan.
- Beat together the eggs, milk, nutmeg and salt and pepper and pour into the pan.
- Bake for 35–40 minutes until firm and golden.

Dairy free option

- Replace milk with 2 additional egg whites.

Recipe information
Serves: 4
Preparation time: 25 minutes
Cooking time: 1 hour

FRITTATA

5 egg whites
10 whole eggs
1 clove garlic
2 onions, chopped
2 tsp mixed herbs
salt and pepper
100g mushrooms, sliced
200g (7 oz) zucchini, sliced
200g (7 oz) asparagus spears (5 cm/2 inch)
1 small sweet potato

- Lightly beat whole eggs and egg whites.
- Sauté garlic and onion in a little stock or water.
- Add sweet potato and cook for 5 minutes.
- Add vegetables and herbs and cook for 3 minutes.
- Place vegetables in ovenproof dish (pan). Pour over egg mix and bake in 200°C (400°F) oven for 45–60 minutes.
- Test with a skewer.

Recipe information
Serves: 10–12
Preparation time: 20 minutes
Cooking time: 1 hour

VEGIE STACK WITH BASIL AND TOMATO SAUCE

2 eggplants
2 sweet potatoes
2 zucchinis
2 red capsicums (bell peppers)
500g (1.1lb) mushrooms
tomato and basil sauce to serve (see recipe page 275)
1 bunch fresh basil

- Slice all vegetables lengthwise approximately ½ cm (¼ inch) thick.
- Char grill all the vegetables on both sides on a hot plate or barbecue until tender.
- Layer vegetables in a stack on individual plates.
- Pour over the tomato and basil sauce and drizzle around the plate.
- Garnish with whole leaves of basil.

Tofu Stack

500g (1.1lb) firm tofu
- Slice tofu into 1 cm (½ inch) thick pieces lengthwise.
- Char grill with vegetables on both sides until brown.
- Layer in between vegetables as above.

Recipe information
Serves: 4–6
Preparation time: 10 minutes
Cooking time: 15 minutes

MAIN MEALS

POACHED CHICKEN WITH BUTTER BEANS, TOMATO, CHILLI AND BASIL

500g butter beans, soaked overnight or equivalent canned
  (2 × 400g/14 oz)

2kg (4.4 lb) medium ripe plum tomatoes, or 2 × 400g (14 oz)
  canned

1 large bunch of basil, roughly chopped

1 medium fresh red chilli pepper, deseeded and finely
  chopped

3 tbsp red wine vinegar

2 tsp extra virgin olive oil

sea salt and cracked pepper

4 poached chicken fillets

- Rinse the soaked beans and cover with water.
- Add 1 tomato, bring to the boil, cover the pan and simmer for about 1½ hours or until tender.
- Blanch the remaining tomatoes, skin, deseed and roughly chop.
- Alternatively use tinned tomatoes.
- Place tomatoes in a bowl and add the basil, chilli pepper, vinegar and oil and mix until combined.
- Drain the cooked butter beans (discard the tomato cooked with them) and gently stir them into the tomato marinade.
- Shred chicken fillets and add to the mix and gently combine.
- Serve warm or cold.

Recipe information
Serves: 4
Preparation time: 30 minutes
Cooking time: 90 minutes

APRICOT CHICKEN

6 chicken breasts, skin removed
425ml (15 oz) can natural apricot nectar
1½ tbsp (2 tbsp) curry powder
425g (15 oz) can apricot halves in natural juice, drained
¼ cup low fat natural yoghurt

- Preheat the oven to 180°C (350°F).
- Place the chicken breasts in an ovenproof pan.
- Place the apricot nectar and curry powder in a bowl and mix together until well combined.
- Pour the mixture over the chicken.
- Bake, covered, for 50 minutes, then add the apricot halves and bake, uncovered, for a further 5 minutes.
- Stir in the yoghurt just before serving.
- Serve with basmati or long grain rice to soak up the juices and steamed broccoli.

Recipe information
Serves: 4–6
Preparation time: 10 minutes
Cooking time: 1 hour

CHICKEN CACCATOIRE

1kg skinless chicken fillets
1 red capsicum
1 Spanish onion
100g button mushrooms
1 small broccoli
1 large can diced tomatoes (800g/1.8 lb)
1 tbsp tomato paste
4 sprigs oregano, chopped
1 stem basil, chopped
½ cup red wine
12 pitted olives
1 clove garlic, crushed (minced)

- Trim and dice chicken.
- Brown chicken on grill or in frying pan, remove and set aside.
- Deseed capsicum and chop into 1½ cm (½ inch) squares.
- Chop onion into chunky squares.
- Remove mushroom stems and clean.
- Cut broccoli into flowerets. Trim stalks and chop these into squares.
- Place chicken and wine into a large pot (pan). Bring to the boil adding garlic and vegetables.
- Next add canned tomatoes, olives and tomato paste.
- Simmer for about 7–8 minutes and add basil and oregano.
- Serve with basmati or long grain rice and/or extra steamed vegetables.

Vegetarian option

- Substitute chicken with tofu.

Recipe information

Serves: 4–6

Preparation time: 15–20 minutes

Cooking time: 25–30 minutes

CHICKEN CURRY

1kg skinless diced chicken fillets
2 tbsp curry powder
1 large sweet potato
1 large onion
1 clove of garlic
½ cauliflower flowerets
2 cups chicken stock
1 tbsp ground cumin
1 cup coriander (cilantro), chopped including roots
1 tsp fresh ginger, chopped
1 bay leaf
2 tsp tahini

- Coat diced chicken fillet in curry powder.
- Seal chicken in hot pan with a small amount of peanut or sesame oil, put aside.
- Sauté onion, garlic, tahini, cumin and ginger in a small amount of chicken stock.
- Add sweet potato and cook for 2–3 minutes.
- Add remaining stock, cauliflower, bay leaf and chicken.
- Cook for a further 30–40 minutes until chicken is cooked.
- Add coriander (cilantro) just before serving.
- Serve with basmati or long grain rice and pappadams.

Tip

- Evenly distribute pappadams on microwave plate and cook on high for 60 seconds until crisp.

> ***Recipe information***
> Serves: 4-6
> Preparation time: 30 minutes
> Cooking time: 30 minutes

STIR-FRIED CHICKEN WITH SNOWPEAS (SUGAR SNAP PEAS) AND MACADAMIAS

1kg (2.2 lb) chicken fillet
1 tbsp sesame oil
300g (10.6 oz) snow peas (sugar snap peas), sliced
  diagonally
½ cup crushed unroasted macadamias
2 tbsp yellow box honey
2 tbsp tamari
coriander (cilantro), chopped
vermicelli noodles

- Trim chicken of all fat and dice into bite size pieces.
- Cook chicken pieces in sesame oil for approximately 6 minutes.
- Add snow peas (sugar snap peas) and cook 3 minutes.
- Add macadamias, honey and tamari and stir-fry until chicken is cooked.
- Prepare noodles according to packet instructions.
- Place a pile of noodles on each plate, top with stir-fry and scatter with coriander (cilantro).

Recipe information
Serves: 4
Preparation time: 10 minutes
Cooking time: 15 minutes

CRUNCHY PECAN CHICKEN

4 small chicken breast fillets, skin removed

2 tbsp yellow box honey

2 tbsp Dijon mustard

1 cup pecans

2 tbsp dry rye breadcrumbs (made from stale 100% rye bread)

½ cup chopped fresh chives

- Preheat oven to hot (220°C/425°F).
- Trim the chicken and place in a 20 × 30cm (8 × 12 in) shallow baking tin with 2 tbsp of water.
- Place the honey and mustard in a bowl and mix together well.
- Place the pecans, breadcrumbs and chives in a food processor, season with salt and freshly ground pepper and process on high until the mixture is roughly chopped and comes together.
- Spread the honey mustard mixture over the chicken breasts then firmly press on the pecan crumbs with your fingers.
- Bake for 15–20 minutes, or until the chicken is cooked and the crumbs are golden brown.
- Serve with a green or rocket salad.

Recipe information

Serves: 4

Preparation time: 15 minutes

Cooking time: 15 minutes

TANDOORI CHICKEN AND SULTANA RICE

1 cup natural yoghurt
juice of 1 lemon
3 tbsp tandoori paste
8 chicken drumsticks or 4 skinless chicken breasts
1 cup red wine
2 cups basmati or long grain rice
½ cup sultanas
sea salt and freshly ground black pepper
natural yoghurt, extra, for serving
4 tbsp coriander (cilantro), roughly chopped
¼ cup toasted almond slivers

- Remove skin from drumsticks and trim all visible fat.
- Mix together the yoghurt, lemon juice and tandoori paste until well combined.
- Coat the chicken in the mixture.
- Place in a deep baking dish and bake for 20 minutes.
- Pour the red wine over the chicken and bake for a further 20 minutes, or until cooked through.
- While chicken is baking, cook the rice in boiling salted water until tender. Strain. Stir through the sultanas.
- To serve – spoon a round bed of sultana rice onto each plate. Sit two drumsticks or one fillet on the rice and spoon over some pan juices. Season. Top the chicken with a dollop of natural yoghurt and sprinkle with coriander (cilantro) and toasted almonds.

Recipe information
Serves: 4
Preparation time: 20 minutes
Cooking time: 40 minutes

CHICKEN BURGERS

1kg lean chicken breast mince
1 large leek
1 large zucchini
⅓ cup mustard seeds
⅓ cup Dijon mustard
handful coriander (cilantro) leaves
1 egg

- Place chicken mince in a large bowl. Cover and leave in refrigerator.
- Grate zucchini and leek and cook in hot frying pan until soft, drain well and leave to cool.
- Thoroughly wash coriander (cilantro) leaves and remove roots.
- Chop leaves and add to mince along with mustard and mustard seeds.
- Mix in cooled leek and zucchini then egg and mix thoroughly.
- Using ½ cup measure, make round patties and refrigerate for 1 hour.
- Cook on a grill at a medium heat for 4–5 minutes on each side or until firm.
- Alternatively bake in moderate oven for 20–25 minutes.

Serving suggestions

- Use in sandwiches or rolls with your favourite fillings.
- Serve with salad or vegetables for a light dinner.
- Serve with basmati rice, salsa and salad.
- Eat individually as a protein snack.

Recipe information
Makes: approximately 10–12 burgers
Preparation time: 30 minutes
Cooking time: 25 minutes

SWEET AND SOUR CHINESE TURKEY

500g (1.1lb) boneless, skinless turkey breasts
2 tbsp lemon juice
5 tbsp orange juice
4 celery sticks (stalks)
2 firm tomatoes
8–10 radishes
½ Chinese cabbage
1 large green pepper (bell pepper), cored and seeded
150ml (¾ cup) chicken stock
1 tbsp soy sauce/tamari
1 tbsp yellow box honey
orange rind (zest), to garnish

- Cut the turkey breast into thin strips. Marinate in the lemon and orange juices for 30 minutes.
- Slice the celery, tomatoes, radishes, Chinese cabbage and green pepper into julienne pieces.
- Roughly chop tomatoes.
- Heat a little stock in a large non-stick pan or wok.
- Drain the turkey and reserve the marinade.
- Fry the turkey in the pan until nearly cooked.
- Add the vegetables and tomatoes and heat for 2–3 minutes.
- Blend the chicken stock with the marinade, add the soy sauce and honey.
- Pour this mixture over the ingredients in the pan and stir until thickened.
- Serve immediately with basmati or long grain rice or vermicelli noodles and garnish with orange rind (zest).

Vegetarian option

• Substitute turkey with tofu.

Recipe information
Serves: 4
Preparation time: 15 minutes, plus marinating
Cooking time: 8 minutes

OSSO BUCCO

4 large veal shanks (approx. 700g/1.5 lb each)
2 carrots, diced
2 large onions, diced
3 sticks (stalks) celery, diced
2 cloves garlic, crushed (minced)
salt and pepper
2 × 400g (14 oz) cans whole, peeled tomatoes
½ cup of red wine
430ml (1½ cups) beef stock
1 tsp dry basil
1 tsp thyme
1 bay leaf
1 small strip of lemon zest
3 tsp parsley, chopped

- Sauté carrots, onions, celery and garlic in a small amount of beef stock until tender.
- Grill veal shanks until sealed on the outside in a dish (pan) suitable for stove top and oven.
- Add tomatoes, wine, stock, basil, thyme, bay leaf and lemon zest to vegetables.
- Bring to the boil and season with salt and pepper.
- Pour vegetable sauce over the shanks, cover and bake in a moderate oven for 1½ hours or until veal is tender.
- Stir through chopped parsley.
- Serve with warm soaked bulgur wheat or wild rice and steamed greens.

Recipe information
Serves: 6–8
Preparation time: 20 minutes
Cooking time: 90 minutes

BOLOGNAISE SAUCE

1kg (2.2 lb) lean beef mince
1 medium onion
1 clove garlic, crushed (minced)
1 cup water or stock
½ bunch fresh oregano
800g (1.8 lb) diced canned or fresh tomatoes
½ cup tomato paste
1 cup red wine
2 bay leaves

- In a large pot cook the mince beef until brown.
- While cooking, break the meat apart with a potato masher until the beef is in small pieces.
- When the mince is ready drain off any excess fat and place pot back on the heat.
- Add onions and garlic to pot then add water or stock and cook until onions are soft.
- Add wine and stir until simmering.
- Add drained mince, tomatoes, tomato paste and bay leaves, stir well.
- Bring to the boil then reduce heat to a simmer. Leave to simmer for 1 hour stirring occasionally.
- Add oregano just at the end.
- Serve with:
  - cooked pasta for lunch.
  - steamed vegetables for dinner.

Recipe information
Serves: 4–6
Preparation time: 30 minutes
Cooking time: 1½ hours

STIR-FRIED BEEF WITH PEPPERS (BELL PEPPERS)

2 tsp sesame oil
1 onion, thinly sliced
1 large garlic clove, cut into thin strips
500g (1.1lb) fillet steak, cut into thin strips
1 red pepper (bell pepper), cored, deseeded and julienned
1 green pepper (bell pepper), cored, deseeded and julienned
1 tbsp tamari
2 tbsp dry sherry
1 tbsp rosemary, chopped
salt and pepper
bok choy to serve
long grain brown rice, to serve (optional)

- Heat the sesame oil in a non-stick frying pan or wok and stir-fry the onion and garlic for 2 minutes.
- Add the strips of beef and stir-fry briskly until evenly browned on all sides and almost tender.
- Add the peppers and stir-fry for a further 2 minutes.
- Add the tamari, sherry, salt and pepper and rosemary and stir-fry for a further 1–2 minutes.
- Serve immediately with brown rice and/or steamed bok choy.

Recipe information
Serves: 4
Preparation time: 15 minutes
Cooking time: about 10 minutes

STEAK WITH TOMATO AND RED ONION SALSA

500g tomatoes (about 4 medium sized)
1 Spanish onion, finely chopped
¼ bunch parsley, leaves finely chopped
¼ bunch basil, leaves finely chopped
25ml (1½ tbsp) balsamic vinegar
2 tsp extra virgin olive oil
sea salt and cracked black pepper
1 tsp olive oil, extra
4 steaks (sirloin), about 200g (7 oz) each

- Drop the tomatoes into a pot of boiling water for about one minute or until the skin starts to lift. Remove with a slotted spoon and place in iced water to cool. Remove the tomatoes, peel, cut in half and scoop out the seeds with a spoon. Dice tomatoes.
- In a large bowl, combine chopped tomatoes, onion, parsley, basil, vinegar and olive oil. Mix well and season to taste. Set aside.
- Season the steaks on both sides. Heat the extra olive oil in a heavy-bottomed pan over a high heat. Once the oil is hot, add the steaks. Cook for 2–3 minutes then turn and cook a further 2–3 minutes (for medium rare; cook for longer if desired) and brown the sides as well.
- Remove and rest for four minutes on a wire rack in a warm place.
- Serve the steaks with a few spoonfuls of salsa.

Recipe information
Serves: 4
Preparation time: 20 minutes
Cooking time: 10 minutes

MEXICAN BEEF BURGERS

1kg beef mince
1 large onion, diced
1 tsp turmeric
1 tsp cumin
1 tsp hot paprika
½ tsp chilli powder
½ tsp cayenne pepper
1 egg
1 tbsp balsamic vinegar
½ cup tomato paste

- Combine all ingredients in a large bowl and mix thoroughly.
- Using a ½ cup measure scoop patties out and set aside to rest for 45 minutes to 1 hour (this will allow patties to hold together better when cooking, but this step is not compulsory).
- Once rested, cook burgers on a hot grill, barbecue or in a pan for 4–5 minutes each side.
- Alternatively, burgers can be baked in an oven (200°C/390°F) for 25 minutes or until cooked through.

Serving options

- Use in sandwiches or rolls with your favourite fillings.
- Serve with salad or vegetables for a light dinner.
- Serve with rice and vegetables.
- Eat individually as a protein snack.

Recipe information
Makes: approximately 10–12 burgers
Preparation time: 20 minutes
Cooking time: 30 minutes

LAMB CUTLETS AND SWEET POTATO MASH

12 lamb cutlets (3 per serve)
1 cup balsamic vinegar
¼ cup tomato paste
2 cloves garlic, crushed (minced)
6 sprigs fresh or 2 tbsp dried rosemary

- Combine vinegar, garlic, tomato paste and rosemary.
- Pour over cutlets and mix well.
- Leave to marinate for one hour or overnight.
- Heat grill or pan to high heat. Cook cutlets for 3–4 minutes on each side until pink in the centre.
- Serve with sweet potato mash (see recipe) and green beans.

Recipe information
Serves: 4
Preparation time: 10 minutes
Cooking time: 10 minutes

LAMB CASSEROLE

1kg diced lamb
½ bunch silver beet
1 cauliflower
500g (1.1 lb) green beans
500g (1.1 lb) sweet potato
¼ cup tomato paste
1 cup red wine
2 tbsp paprika
1 tsp chilli powder
1 tsp garam marsala
1 tsp garlic, crushed (minced)
1 tbsp oregano

- Trim, slice and wash silver beet.
- Cut cauliflower into flowerets.
- Top and tail beans.
- Peel and cube sweet potato.
- Seal lamb on hot grill or in frying pan.
- Mix together wine, tomato paste, herbs and spices in a bowl.
- Place lamb and sauce into a large pot and simmer on low heat for 35-40 minutes or until meat is almost tender.
- Add sweet potato and cook for 5 minutes.
- Add remaining vegetables and stir. Cover and cook for another 10 minutes or until vegetables are just crunchy.
- Serve in deep bowls.

Vegetarian option

- Substitute lamb with cooked lentils or chickpeas (garbanzo beans).

Recipe information
Serves: 4–6
Preparation time: 40 minutes
Cooking time: 60 minutes

CHINESE PORK WITH BAMBOO SHOOTS

300g (10.6 oz) lean pork, shredded
1 small Chinese cabbage, shredded
1 tbsp coarsely chopped hazelnuts
250g (8.8 oz) canned bamboo shoots sliced, drained with
  juices reserved
2 tbsp tamari
1 tsp curry powder
pinch of chilli powder
salt and pepper
extra tamari, to serve (optional)
extra cooked cabbage to serve

- Heat a non-stick frying pan or wok, add the pork and stir-fry quickly until lightly browned – season with salt and pepper.
- Add the cabbage, hazelnuts and a few tablespoons of the liquid from the can of bamboo shoots.
- Cook, stirring, for about 5 minutes.
- Add the bamboo shoots, reserving some to garnish, tamari, curry powder, and chilli powder, mixing well.
- Cook gently for a further 10 minutes.
- Serve immediately with cooked cabbage dressed with extra tamari and garnish with the reserved bamboo shoots.

Vegetarian option

- Substitute pork with firm tofu.

Recipe information
Serves: 4
Preparation time: 15 minutes
Cooking time: 20 minutes

MUSTARD SWORDFISH

4 swordfish steaks

2 tbsp low-salt soy sauce or tamari

2 tbsp lemon juice

2 tsp grated, fresh ginger

2 tbsp wholegrain mustard

- Combine soy sauce, mustard, ginger and lemon juice in a bowl.
- Drizzle mixture over fish steaks and grill under medium heat for 3–4 minutes.
- Turn fish over, drizzle mixture over other side, and grill for another 3–4 minutes or more depending on the thickness of the steaks.
- Serve with salad.

Recipe information

Serves: 4

Preparation time: 10 minutes

Cooking time: 8 minutes

MEDITERRANEAN SALMON

200g (7 oz) green beans
20 small cherry tomatoes
1–2 handfuls of black olives (approximately 15)
1 tsp extra virgin olive oil
salt and pepper
4 × 225g (8 oz) thick salmon fillets steaks, with or without
  skin
2 lemons
1 handful of fresh basil
12 anchovy fillets

- Top and tail (clean) the green beans, blanch until tender and drain.
- Put in a bowl with the cherry tomatoes and stoned (pitted) olives. Toss with olive oil, and pepper.
- Wash and dry salmon fillets and squeeze the juice of ½ a lemon over the fillets.
- Season with salt and pepper.
- Toss the basil into the green beans, olives and tomatoes and place at one end of a roasting dish (pan). Place the fish at the other end of the dish.
- Lay the anchovies over the green beans and roast all ingredients in a hot oven for 10 minutes.
- Remove from oven.
- Serve ¼ of bean mixture with one salmon fillet on top.
- Garnish with lemon wedges.

Recipe information
Serves: 4
Preparation time: 10 minutes
Cooking time: 10 minutes

TOMATOES, OLIVE AND BASIL INFUSED FISH

4 John Dory fillets, scaled (each about 225g/8 oz)
salt and pepper
2 glasses dry white wine

Marinade
1 handful of black olives, stoned (pitted)
1 clove of garlic, peeled and finely chopped
½ small dried red chilli pepper
1 handful of fresh basil or marjoram, roughly chopped
1 tsp extra virgin olive oil
20 cherry tomatoes, halved
1 lemon

- Put the olives into a bowl with the garlic, chilli, herbs and oil.
- Add the cherry tomatoes and leave about ½ hour.
- Add lemon juice to taste.
- On a piece of foil place a quarter of the marinated ingredients with one John Dory fillet on top.
- Season fish with salt and pepper.
- Fold over the foil and seal two sides.
- Add ½ cup of the white wine per pocket and seal the remaining side of the foil.
- Repeat the process for the remaining fillets.
- Bake in a hot oven for approximately 10 minutes, remove from oven and allow to stand for 3–4 minutes without opening the bag.
- To serve, place an unopened bag on each plate.
- Serve with steamed greens.

Recipe information
Serves: 4
Preparation time: 45 minutes
Cooking time: 15 minutes

VEGETARIAN MAIN MEALS

LENTIL BOLOGNAISE SAUCE

½ cup uncooked brown or green lentils or equivalent tinned
1 medium onion, finely chopped
2½ cups diced mushrooms
400g (14 oz) can chopped tomatoes
2 tbsp tomato paste
2 tbsp water
2 cloves garlic, crushed (minced)
½ tsp dried marjoram
1 small bay leaf
1 tbsp tamari
chopped parsley

- Place lentils in a saucepan of water. Bring uncovered to the boil, skim, cover and simmer for about 30 minutes or until soft. Drain.
- Heat the water in a saucepan and soften the onion and garlic for 4–5 minutes.
- Add mushrooms, cooked lentils, marjoram and bay leaf and cook for 10 minutes.
- Stir in tomatoes and tomato paste.
- Cover and cook for 20–25 minutes.
- Remove bay leaf and mash the lentil mix to a sauce consistency.
- Season with tamari and stir through parsley.
- Serve with pasta, as a side dish or pour over steamed vegetables.

Recipe information
Serves: 4
Preparation time: 40 minutes
Cooking time: 25 minutes

BEST EVER CANNELLONI WITH TOMATO BASIL SAUCE

Cannelloni
1 packet rye mountain bread (flat bread)
1kg sweet potatoes
1 250g (8.8 oz) tub of smooth, low fat ricotta cheese
250g (8.8 oz) baby spinach leaves
Sauce
2 × 400g (14 oz) cans diced tomatoes
1 bunch of basil
1 large onion diced
1 clove garlic, crushed (minced)
⅓ cup tomato paste

- Prepare tomato sauce (see below).
- Peel and dice sweet potato. Place in a pot and cover with water. Bring to the boil then simmer for 15–18 minutes or until potato is soft.
- When ready strain, and while still hot add ricotta cheese and mash until smooth.
- Julienne baby spinach and mix well into potato mix.
- Using a piping bag without a nozzle, pipe about a 20 cent piece (1 inch) diameter amount of the potato mix along the longest edge of the mountain (flat) bread, grain side down.
- Gently roll up the bread, cut in half.
- Serve immediately with tomato and basil sauce poured over the top.
- Serve 3 halves per person.

Tomato basil sauce

- Add diced onion and garlic to a medium pot, cook on a moderate heat until onions are soft.

- Add canned tomatoes and tomato paste. Bring to the boil and then reduce to a simmer.
- Simmer gently until cannelloni is prepared.
- Just before serving, stir torn basil leaves through sauce and ladle over cannelloni.

Recipe information

Serves: 5

Preparation time: 20 minutes

Cooking time: 30 minutes

ROAST CAPSICUM, ZUCCHINI AND ANCHOVY ORECCHIETTE

2 red capsicums (bell peppers), roasted and peeled (see
  Greek Salad recipe page 290)
2 cloves garlic
¼ cup vegetable stock
cracked pepper
8–10 anchovy fillets, roughly chopped
2 tbsp oregano leaves
3 zucchinis, sliced and roasted
500g orecchiette (or your favourite pasta)

- Prepare capsicum and zucchini.
- Place capsicum and capsicum juices, garlic and vegetable stock in a blender and process to make a smooth sauce.
- Transfer to a saucepan and bring to the boil, adding pepper to taste.
- Add anchovies, oregano and zucchini and heat through.
- Meanwhile, cook pasta in plenty of boiling salted water and then drain.
- Toss pasta with capsicum sauce and serve with rocket salad.

Recipe information
Serves: 6–8
Preparation time: 20 minutes
Cooking time: 25 minutes

VEGETARIAN LASAGNA

12 fresh lasagne sheets
800g (1.8 lb) can diced tomatoes
¼ cup tomato paste
1 medium zucchini
1 eggplant
1 red capsicum
1 medium onion
200g (7 oz) button mushrooms
1 clove chopped garlic
1 tbsp mixed herbs
¼ cup red wine
150g (5.3 oz) low fat cottage cheese

Centre filling
1 medium sweet potato
250g (8.8 oz) low fat ricotta cheese
100g baby spinach (washed)

- Bring a large pot of water to the boil for the pasta sheets, cook sheets until al dente, cool, and leave to the side.
- Peel and cook the sweet potato, drain then mash with ricotta while still hot, leave to cool.
- Chop vegetables into 1cm (½ inch) pieces.
- In a medium size pot, add a little water and cook onions and garlic until soft.
- Add red wine, vegetables, tomatoes and tomato paste.
- Bring to the boil adding herbs, reduce heat and simmer for half an hour.
- Using a suitable dish (pan), cover bottom with cooked lasagne sheets.
- Ladle a thin layer of the tomato mix onto the lasagne sheets, then cover with more lasagne sheets.
- Spread the potato mix on top, cover this with the spinach leaves, another layer of pasta and the remainder of the tomato sauce and finish with a layer of pasta.

- Mix cottage cheese with mixed herbs and cover the top layer of pasta.
- Cover and refrigerate until cool and set.
- Reheat in low oven for approximately 25 minutes.

Recipe information

Serves: 6–8

Preparation time: 40 minutes

Cooking time: 40 minutes

CHICKPEA (GARBANZO BEAN) AND SWEET POTATO CURRY

450g (1 lb) cooked chickpeas (garbanzo beans) or
   equivalent tinned
2 sweet potatoes
400g can diced tomatoes
1½ tsp cumin seeds
1½ tsp mustard seeds
1½ tsp tumeric powder
1 onion finely chopped
2 cloves garlic finely chopped (minced)
1 tsp chilli pepper (or sambal oelek)
1 coriander (cilantro) plant (leaves, roots and stalks)
1 tsp salt
yoghurt to serve

- Peel sweet potato and cut into cubes.
- Steam for 3 minutes, should still be firm.
- Roast mustard seeds and cumin seeds in a frying pan until fragrant.
- Add turmeric, onion, garlic, chilli and ½ coriander (cilantro) with a little water to prevent sticking.
- When onion is cooked add sweet potato, chickpeas (garbanzo beans), tomatoes, salt and cook for 10 minutes.
- Serve with steamed greens and/or basmati or long grain rice.
- Garnish with a dollop of natural yoghurt and coriander (cilantro) leaves.

Recipe information
Serves: 4
Preparation time: 15 minutes
Cooking time: 20 minutes

LENTIL BURGERS

2 cups of brown lentils or equivalent tinned
1 large brown or Spanish onion
1 cup grated carrot
1 cup grated zucchini
1 cup cooked basmati or long grain rice
2 cloves of garlic
salt and pepper
2 cups vegetable stock

- Cook lentils in plenty of water until softened; drain.
- Sauté diced onion and garlic in a small amount of water.
- Add lentils and 2 cups of stock.
- Cook on low until lentils have softened and absorbed some of the stock, approximately 20 minutes.
- Allow to cool.
- In a large bowl combine cooked rice, carrot, zucchini and lentil mixture (mixture should be fairly dry).
- Knead and season well with salt and pepper.
- Form into balls and place on a non stick baking tray (sheet) in a moderate oven (180°C/350°F).
- Bake for 30 minutes or until brown.
- Serve with salad or vegetables.

Recipe information
Serves: 24 burgers
Preparation time: 20 minutes
Cooking time: 60 minutes

SNACKS AND DESSERTS

ENERGY BALLS

½ cup finely chopped prunes

½ cup finely chopped dried apple

½ cup finely chopped dried apricots

1 tbsp yellow box honey

½ cup finely chopped pecans

½ cup ground almonds

- Mix ingredients thoroughly together.
- Roll into small balls.
- Store in refrigerator in airtight container.

Recipe information

Serves: 15–25 balls (depending on size)

Preparation time: 15–20 minutes

HUMBLE CRUMBLE

6 Granny Smith apples (green apples)
1 cup brown rice flour
1 cup rolled millet (or whole rolled oats)
1 cup coconut
rind (zest) of one lemon
2 tsp cinnamon
¼ cup yellow box honey

- Thinly slice the apple and/or other fruit.
- Arrange fruit in a shallow, ovenproof dish (pan).
- Combine the rice flour, millet, coconut, rind and cinnamon and mix thoroughly.
- Warm the honey and add to the mixture, stirring to make a crumble.
- Spread the crumble carefully over the fruit.
- Bake in a 180°C (350°F) oven for approximately 15 minutes or until lightly browned and crunchy.

Variations

- Substitute apple with 4 pears and 12 dried apricots.
- Add ½ bunch washed and chopped rhubarb to apple mix.

Recipe information
Serves: 4
Preparation time: 10–15 minutes
Cooking time: 15–20 minutes

GRANOLA CAKE

175g (6 oz) natural muesli (granola)
175g (6 oz) sultanas
2 tbsp yellow box honey
250ml (1 cup) 100% apple juice
2 cooking (green) apples, cored and grated
175g (6 oz) wholemeal (whole wheat) flour
3 tsp baking powder
11 walnut halves

- Preheat oven to 180°C (350°F).
- Place the muesli (granola), sultanas, honey and apple juice in a mixing bowl and leave to soak for 30 minutes.
- Add the apple and sift in the baking powder and flour.
- Fold ingredients together.
- Turn into a lined and greased 18cm (7 in) round cake tin and arrange the walnuts around the edge.
- Bake in a preheated oven for 1½ hours, or until a skewer inserted into the centre comes out clean.
- Leave the cake in the tin for a few minutes, then turn out onto a wire rack to cool.

Recipe information
Serves: 8–10
Preparation time: 15 minutes, plus soaking
Cooking time: 1½ hours

LUNCHBOX LOAF

1¼ cups water
¾ cup chopped dried or fresh dates
1 cup chopped walnuts
1 tsp mixed spice
1 tbsp honey (optional)
¾ cup soy flour
¾ cup brown rice flour
1 tsp bicarb soda (baking soda)
2 tsp cream of tartar
2 tsp lemon juice

- Preheat oven to 180°C (350°F).
- Add water, dates, walnuts and spices to a pot.
- Heat gently and bring to the boil.
- Remove from heat and stir in honey.
- Leave to cool.
- When cool fold through flours, bicarb soda (baking soda) and cream of tartar.
- Add lemon juice and mix.
- Pour into a lightly greased loaf tin (loaf pan) and bake in oven for 30 minutes or until firm.
- Allow to cool.

Variation

- Glace with sugar-free jam, warmed on stove and spread over loaf.

Recipe information
Serves: 6
Preparation time: 20–30 minutes
Cooking time: 30-40 minutes

SMART LEMON TART

Base

½ cup brown rice flour
½ cup rolled millet
½ cup coconut
4 tbsp water

- Preheat oven to 180°C (350°F).
- Combine flour, millet and coconut.
- Mix with water and press onto a lightly greased pie plate.
- Do not bake before filling.

Filling

3 eggs, lightly beaten
½ cup lemon juice
2½ tbsp yellow box honey
rind (zest) of 1 lemon
2 apples, peeled and grated
cinnamon

- Blend eggs, lemon juice, honey and rind (zest).
- Pour into pie shell.
- Sprinkle with grated apple and cinnamon.
- Bake in oven for approximately 30 minutes.
- Allow to cool and refrigerate.
- Serve with fresh berries.

Recipe information
Serves: 4–5
Preparation time: 20–30 minutes
Cooking time: 30 minutes

AWESOME APPLE PIE

Base

½ cup coconut
½ cup ground pecans
1 cup ground almonds

- Combine ingredients and press over pie plate.
- Bake blind in moderate oven for 10 minutes.

Filling

6 Granny Smith (green) apples, peeled and chopped
6 cloves cloves
1 tbsp yellow box honey
stick cinnamon
water
strip lemon rind (zest), finely chopped
1 tsp ground cinnamon

- Cover base of saucepan with water.
- Add apples, cloves, honey, cinnamon stick and lemon rind (zest).
- Gently heat and simmer until apples are soft.
- Remove cinnamon stick.
- Pour into pie crust (pie shell) and dust with cinnamon.
- Bake in moderate oven (180°C/350°F) for 20–30 minutes.

Recipe information
Serves: 4–6
Preparation time: 20–30 minutes
Cooking time: 30–40 minutes

RICOTTA CHEESECAKE

Base

½ cup brown rice flour
½ cup rolled millet
½ cup coconut
4 tbsp water

- Preheat oven to 180°C (350°F).
- Combine grains and coconut.
- Mix water and press onto a lightly greased pie plate.
- Do not bake before filling.

Filling

3 cups low fat ricotta cheese or a combination of low fat
  ricotta and cottage cheese
4 eggs
¾ cup natural yoghurt
½ cup yellow box honey
⅓ cup lemon juice
rind (zest) one lemon
few drops pure vanilla
fruit to serve

- Blend cheeses, eggs, yoghurt, honey, lemon juice and rind, and vanilla with an electric beater until smooth.
- Pour onto crust (shell) and bake for 15–20 minutes or until set.
- Cool then refrigerate.
- Once cool, top with passionfruit, strawberries and/or kiwifruit.
- Serve immediately.

Recipe information

Serves: 8

Preparation time: 20–30 minutes

Cooking time: 20 minutes

STRAWBERRY SORBET

2 punnets strawberries (500g)

½ cup 100% apple juice (no added sugar)

½ cup water

¼ cup yellow box honey

- Blend all ingredients with an electric beater.
- Freeze in a suitable container.
- Before serving, remove from freezer and allow sufficient softening to permit blending.
- Blend until mixture resembles soft ice-cream.
- Ladle icy mixture into open champagne glasses or small dessert bowls.
- Top with whole strawberry.

Recipe information

Serves: 4

Preparation time: 15–20 minutes (plus freezing time)

Conclusion

Well, it's been quite a journey. I thank you for having enough faith in me to get to the end of this book. That is of course unless you skipped to the last chapter to see how it ends!

I will tell you how it ends. The truth is, it doesn't end. This is the beginning of the rest of your life. How this journey turns out is 100 percent in your hands.

The plan I have outlined is not the only path to a long and happy life but it is a tried and tested one.

You have a fantastic opportunity to take control of your life. The way you think, the way you behave, the way you react to certain situations, the effort you make to change limiting behaviours, the consistent approach you take, the way you feel about yourself and the faith you have will determine the final outcome.

Here are the facts in black and white:

- You are in control of your destiny.

- If you can control your energy levels (blood sugar levels) you will be able to achieve more in your career, personal and sporting life than you ever thought possible.

- With the knowledge you now have about Glycemic Index and the importance of eating small regular meals throughout the day, you will be able to create the body you want.

- Long-term changes don't happen quickly. Take the time to learn and change habits that have prevented you from achieving your goals.

- Eating a balance and variety of fresh and natural whole foods, healthy fats, and quality proteins will provide your body with the nutrients it needs for optimal health.

- Supplementing your eating plan with natural, plant-based vitamins, minerals and phytochemicals will enhance your health, happiness and longevity.

- Understanding how to read labels and interpret marketing ploys will help you make wise choices when shopping for food.

- Understand the importance of indulgence and balance when eating and in all areas of your life.

- Include regular exercise in your life.

- Enjoy the process and you will reap the rewards.

- Make a plan and work through it systematically until you have achieved the outcome you desire. Be persistent and consistent.

- Be happy, love yourself and make the most of your time on earth.

I hope you have gained something from this book. If you change only one thing, but that one thing makes your life better, then it has been worthwhile.

Please don't spend anymore time looking for an easy option or a fast fix. From this point and for the rest of your life, take the time to develop a lifestyle that brings you pleasure and enables you to achieve all the things you desire in your world. It is most definitely possible – have faith, the answer is in your hands.

Now go and have a beer or wine and a piece of chocolate and enjoy!

Appendix

Glycemic Index Lists

FOOD	APPROX. GI
Bakery Products – Breads	
Bagel	72
Barley bread – coarse barley kernel	30
Barley flour bread	65–70
Barley flour flat bread	40–50
Barley kernel bread	45
Burgen™ – fruit bread	44
Burgen™ – dark rye	74
Burgen™ – oatbran and honey	31
Burgen™ – soy and linseed	36
Buckwheat bread	47
Country Life – Performax™	38
Fruit and Spice (Buttercup)	54
French white baguette	95
Gluten free	70–80
Helga's™ Classic Seed Loaf	68
Helga's™ Traditional Wholemeal Loaf	70

Lebanese	75
Light rye	68
Middle Eastern flat bread	97
Multigrain	50–60
Oat bran bread (50% oat bran)	44
Pita	57
Ploughman's™ Wholegrain	47
Ploughman's™ Wholemeal	64
Pumpernickel	41
Rice bread	72
Rye kernel	46
Sourdough rye	48
Spelt flour bread	54
Tip Top Holsom's 9 Grain™	43
Turkish bread (white flour)	87
Turkish bread (whole wheat flour)	49
Vogel's™ Honey and Oats	55
Vogel's™ Roggenbrot	59
White bread	70
Wholemeal bread	77
Wonderwhite™	80

Bakery Products – Other

Croissant	67
Crumpet	69
Cupcake	73
English muffin	77
Flan cake	65
Lamington	87
Muffin (cake-style)	45–70
Pancake	67
Pikelet	85
Pound cake	54
Scone	92
Sponge cake	46
Waffle	76

Breakfast Bars

Crunchy Nut Cornflakes™ bar	72
Fibre Plus™ bar	78
Fruity-Bix™ bar	54
K-time Just Right™	72
Rice Bubble Treat™	63
Sustain™	57

Breakfast Cereals

All Bran™ – fruit 'n' oats	39
All Bran™ – high fibre	30
All Bran™ – soy 'n' fibre	33
Bran flakes™	74
Barley porridge	65
Coco pops™	77
Cornflakes™	77
Crunchy Nut Cornflakes™	72
Fibre Plus™	78
Froot Loops™	69
Frosties™	55
Good Start™	68
Golden Wheats™	71
Guardian™	37
Healthwise™ for bowel	66
Healthwise™ for heart	48
Honey Goldies™	72
Honey Rice Bubbles™	77
Honey Smacks™	71
Just Right™	60
Just Right™ Just Grains	62
Komplete™	48
Light-Bix™	70
Muesli – natural	40–50
Mini Wheats™ – whole wheat	58
Mini Wheats™ – blackcurrant	72

Nutrigrain™	66
Oat 'n' Honey Bake™	77
Oat bran (raw)	55
Pop Tarts™	70
Porridge	40–60
Puffed wheat	80
Rice Bubbles™	83
Special K™	54
Soy Tasty™	60
Soytana™	49
Sultana Bran™	73
Sultana Goldies™	65
Sustain™	68
Ultra Bran™	41
Vita Brits™	68
Wheat-Bites™	72
Weetbix™	69
Weetbix™ – high bran	57

Crispbreads and Crackers

Breton	67
Corn thins	87
Jatz™	55
Kavli™	71
Premium™/Saladas™	74
Rice cakes/crackers	87
Ryvita™	69
Sao™	70
Taco shells	68
Vitaweat™	55
Water crackers	78

Dairy Products

Chocolate	45
Custard	35–45

Ice cream	61
Ice cream – low fat	50
Milk – full cream	27
Milk – skim	32
Yoghurt – low fat with sugar	24
Yoghurt – low fat, artificially sweetened	14
Yoghurt – soy, low fat	50

Soy Milk

Full-fat, Calciforte (So Natural™)	36
Full-fat, Original (So Natural™)	44
Reduced-fat, Original (So Natural™)	44

Drinks

Coca Cola®	53
Cordial	66
Fanta®	68
Gatorade®	78
Lucozade®	95
Solo™	58
Sports plus®	74
Sustagen Sport®	43
Up and Go – cocoa malt	43
Up and Go – original	46
Yakult®	46

Drinks Made from Powders

Milo™ – in water	55
Milo™ – in full-fat milk	35
Quik™ – chocolate, in water	53
Quik™ – chocolate, in low-fat milk	41
Quik™ – strawberry, in water	64
Quik™ – strawberry, in low-fat milk	35

Fresh Fruit

Apple	38
Apricot	57
Banana	50–60
Cherries	22
Cantaloupe	65
Grape	46
Grapefruit	25
Kiwifruit	58
Mango	55
Orange	44
Paw paw	58
Peach	42
Pear	38
Pineapple	66
Plum	39
Strawberries	40
Watermelon	72

Dried Fruit

Apple	29
Apricots	30
Dates	103
Figs	61
Prunes	29
Raisins	64
Sultanas	56

Fruit Products

Strawberry jam	51
Strawberry Real Fruit Bars™	90
Tropical Fruity Bitz™	41
Vitari™ frozen dessert	59
Wild Berry Fruity Bitz™	35

Grains

Buckwheat	55
Cornmeal	68
Couscous	69
Millet/maize	71
Oats	42
Pearl barley	25
Semolina	55
Tapioca	70

Rice

Aborio	69
Basmati	57
Calrose white – medium grain	80
Calrose brown	87
Doongara	56
Instant white	87
Instant Doongara	94
Mahatma – long grain	50
Sunbrown quick	80
Sungold	87

Infant Formula and Weaning Foods

Farex™ baby rice	95
Heinz for baby from 4 months	65
Infasoy™	55
Nan-1™	30
S-26™	36

Juice

Apple	40
Carrot	43
Cranberry	52

Grapefruit	48
Orange	53
Pineapple	46
Tomato	38

Honey

Commercial blend Capilano	72
Iron Bark	48
Pure Capilano	58
Red Gum	46
Salvation Jane	64
Stringy Bark	44
Yapunya	52
Yellow Box	35

Legumes

Baked beans	48
Black beans	30
Broad beans	79
Butter beans	31
Chickpeas	34
Haricot beans	38
Kidney beans	27
Lentils – green	37
Lentils – red	26
Lima beans	33
Mung beans	40
Soy beans	20
Split peas	32

Nuts

Almonds	0
Brazil nuts	0
Cashews	22

Hazelnuts	0
Macadamias	0
Peanuts	20
Pecans	0

Pasta

Fettucine	32
Gnocchi	68
Linguine	52
Macaroni	45
Ravioli – meat filled	39
Rice pasta	92
Spaghetti	30–60
Two Minute Noodles®	46
Udon noodles	62
Vermicelli	35

Protein Foods

Beef	0
Eggs	0
Fish	0
Lamb	0
Pork	0
Shellfish	0
Veal	0

Snack Foods

Burger Rings	90
Cashews	22
Corn chips	72
Doughnut	76
Heinz Kids™ Fruit Fingers	61
Jelly Beans	80
Life Savers®	70

Mars Bar®	65
M & Ms® – peanut	62
Nutella®	33
Popcorn	89
Potato crisps	57
Pretzels	83
Real Fruit Bars® (Uncle Toby's)	90
Roll-Ups®	99
Snickers®	41
Twisties™	74
Twix®	44

Sugars

Dextrose	100
Fructose	23
Glucose	100
Lactose	48
Maltose	105
Sucrose	60

Vegetables

Artichokes	0
Avocado	0
Beetroot	64
Bok choy	0
Broccoli	0
Cabbage	0
Capsicum	0
Carrot	49
Cauliflower	0
Celery	0
Cucumber	0
Leafy vegetables	0
Parsnip	97
Peas	48

Potatoes

Desiree	101
Instant mashed	86
New	78
Pontiac	88
Sebago	87
Pumpkin	75
Sweetcorn	55
Sweet potato	50
Yam	51

Supporting Reference

Brand-Miller, J., *The New Glucose Revolution* (2002), Hodder Headline Australia Pty Ltd.

Recipe Index

Index

DAILY FOOD DIARY

DAY . . . . DATE . . /. . /. . .

TIME	QTY	DESCRIPTION	MOOD	ENERGY LEVELS

Water Consumed (glasses)　　　1　2　3　4　5　6　7　8　9　10

Mood	Excellent	Good	Fair	Poor
Energy Levels	Very High	High	Moderate	Low

DAILY FOOD DIARY

DAY . . . . DATE . . /. . /. . .

TIME	QTY	DESCRIPTION	MOOD	ENERGY LEVELS

Water Consumed (glasses)   1   2   3   4   5   6   7   8   9   10

Mood	Excellent	Good	Fair	Poor
Energy Levels	Very High	High	Moderate	Low

DAILY FOOD DIARY

DAY . . . . DATE . . /. . /. . .

TIME	QTY	DESCRIPTION	MOOD	ENERGY LEVELS

Water Consumed (glasses)   1   2   3   4   5   6   7   8   9   10

Mood	Excellent	Good	Fair	Poor
Energy Levels	Very High	High	Moderate	Low

DAILY FOOD DIARY

DAY . . . . DATE . . ./. . ./. . .

TIME	QTY	DESCRIPTION	MOOD	ENERGY LEVELS

Water Consumed (glasses)   1   2   3   4   5   6   7   8   9   10

Mood	Excellent	Good	Fair	Poor
Energy Levels	Very High	High	Moderate	Low

DAILY FOOD DIARY

DAY . . . . DATE . . ./. . ./. . .

TIME	QTY	DESCRIPTION	MOOD	ENERGY LEVELS

Water Consumed (glasses)   1   2   3   4   5   6   7   8   9   10

Mood	Excellent	Good	Fair	Poor
Energy Levels	Very High	High	Moderate	Low

DAILY FOOD DIARY

DAY . . . . DATE . . /. . /. . .

TIME	QTY	DESCRIPTION	MOOD	ENERGY LEVELS

Water Consumed (glasses)   1   2   3   4   5   6   7   8   9   10

Mood	Excellent	Good	Fair	Poor
Energy Levels	Very High	High	Moderate	Low